# Comments on *Paradoxical Relaxation*

David Wise's *Paradoxical Relaxation* is a ground-breaking book, describing principles of relaxation training not part of mainstream methods of relaxation. The insights in this book about the nature and practice of relaxation are profound and can be of enormous benefit to those who struggle with varieties of stress related disorders. *Paradoxical Relaxation* was developed and tested in the work Wise did at Stanford University with Rodney Anderson in the Department of Urology with individuals with pelvic pain and dysfunction. In this needed volume, Dr. Wise presents the method he uses for the treatment of pelvic pain for the larger application of treating anxiety and anxiety-related disorders. The method of *Paradoxical Relaxation*, while discussed as part of the *Wise-Anderson Protocol* in the best-selling book, *A Headache in the Pelvis*, is presented here in a level of detail heretofore unavailable.

*Robert Blum, MD*
*Former Chairman of the Department of Neurosurgery,*
*Marin General Hospital*

This book that David Wise has written on relaxation training clearly is not an abstract rendering of a theoretical position, but the record of lessons personally learned, and here taught. Dr. Wise has distinguished himself by co-developing a successful treatment for chronic pelvic pain syndromes at Stanford University called the *Wise-Anderson Protocol. Paradoxical Relaxation* is a careful exploration of one of the methods of this innovative protocol and a departure from conventional relaxation training for anxiety. Dr. Wise's book is self-revelatory in taking us through his journey to free himself from pelvic pain. This method has been used with his pelvic pain patients over the years and its effectiveness has been documented in published studies. *Paradoxical Relaxation* can be of significant value for those wishing to learn relaxation in order to deal with anxiety and anxiety related disorders.

*Alan Leveton, M.D.*
*Associate Clinical Professor, Pediatrics and Psychiatry (retired)*
*University of California, School of Medicine, San Francisco*

# Paradoxical Relaxation

The theory and practice of
dissolving anxiety by accepting it

David Wise, Ph.D.

Paradoxical Relaxation
The Theory and Practice of
Dissolving Anxiety by Accepting It


National Center for Pelvic Pain Research
P.O. Box 54
Occidental, CA 95465
Toll Free 866-874-2225
Fax 707-874-2335

Cover design by Patricia Lachman

Publisher's Cataloging-in-Publication Data

Wise, David Thomas, 1945-
Paradoxical relaxation : the theory and practice of dissolving anxiety by accepting it / David Wise. -- 1st ed. -- Occidental, CA : National Center for Pelvic Pain Research, ©2010.
p. ; cm.
ISBN: 978-0-9727755-8-8
1. Relaxation--Methodology--Popular works. 2. Anxiety--Prevention--Popular works. 3. Stress management--Popular works. 4. Meditation--Popular works. I. Title.
BF637.R45 W57 2010 2010921180
613.7/92--dc22 1002

2 4 6 8 9 7 5 3

First edition

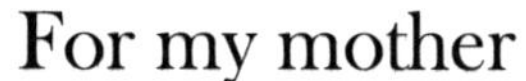

For my mother

# Table of Contents

## Acknowledgements

This acknowledgements page recognizes with gratitude who or what has helped or contributed to this book. When I think about who and what I want to recognize and appreciate as having contributed to this book, I want to make an acknowledgement that you would rarely read in the acknowledgements of a book. I want to acknowledge the contribution of my suffering with pelvic pain and anxiety because without it I believe I never would have even had the interest in learning how to profoundly relax. I want to acknowledge the teachers I have studied with who have devoted themselves to quieting down body and mind. First among these is Edmund Jacobson, the founder of Progressive Relaxation, without whose example and inspiration I would not have written this book. I also wish to thank Helen Morcos for her invaluable help with Progressive Relaxation. I particularly want to acknowledge Walter Blum who has walked the talk of this method more than anyone I have ever known and whose story I have included in these pages. I want to thank John Moses for his keen observations, insights, his helpful suggestions and his invaluable support in communicating the ideas herein contained. I want to acknowledge my meditation teachers and those who have explored different aspects of the world of the psyche, including Alan Leveton, Frederick Perls, Ramana Maharshi, Nisargadatta, Poonja-ji, Koryu Roshi, Suzuki Roshi, Jim Simpkin, Roberto Assagioli, Robert Hall, Byron Katie, Jean Kline, Kathy Harris, Allaudin Mathieu, Mary and Harry Kenney, Ann Dreyfus, Leo Zeff, Richard Miller. I would like to acknowledge and thank friends and family including Harold Wise, June Wise, Fay Nathanson, Brian Nathanson, Larry Nathanson and Helene Korn. Many thanks to my amazing colleagues Rodney Anderson and Tim Sawyer in our remarkable work with pelvic pain. Thanks to Tiaga Liner, Alan and Victoria Dreyfus, Dan and Tara Fink, Frank and Susan Werblin and Elaine Orenberg-Anderson. I particularly want to thank Hilary Garcia, my editor and transcriber, whose patience, good humor, and keen intelligence has been essential in completing this book. I also wish to express my gratitude and appreciation to Patricia Lachman for the beautiful cover of this book that she designed, and to Claudia Fiori, Jennifer Tien and Elliot Isenberg for their excellent editorial help.

# Introduction

Describing how to profoundly relax and the impediments to this noble aspiration is describing the ineffable. It is describing what words cannot quite reach.

In this introduction, I address my dilemma of what to remove in this book that might appear to be repetitive. Words generally can only express one idea at a time. When describing something multi-faceted, words can only describe one facet after another. The second facet has to wait to be described until the words finish describing the first. The second facet might blur into the first, or might be part of explaining the third facet, especially when the subject is as subtle as how to profoundly relax. This blurring may appear repetitive.

At the turn of the $20^{th}$ century, Picasso and the cubists introduced a form of art which attempted to represent all different aspects of an object at once. When depicting a face in profile, Picasso would paint both the eye that was visible and the eye that was not visible in profile on the same plane. It was a fascinating and revolutionary experiment.

Words, however, do not lend themselves to the expression of the whole all at once. In the description of the different facets of *Paradoxical Relaxation,* the description of one facet tends to overlap into others.

I have looked hard at what may appear to be repetitive in this volume. I have decided to err on the side of leaving in some sections that might appear to be similar or repetitive because I hope they will best explain this methodology. I beg the reader's indulgence in my decision to do this.

This book does not have to be read from cover to cover. It can just be opened up and read one paragraph at a time. You can read this book by just reading the subtitles and text boxes or, of course, you can read it in the standard way by reading cover to cover, from beginning to end. Whatever way you may read it, I hope it will be helpful to you in the same way it is to me.

# Chapter 1

***If you want to learn how to relax, you can***

## ***Paradoxical Relaxation* is the practice of entering a sanctuary undisturbed by the world**

Imagine during your day of emails, phone calls, bad news on the television—what Zorba the Greek called 'the catastrophe of our life'—you could say, "Excuse me, I need to spend some time in heaven." Imagine you could walk through a door, close it behind you, and in 15 minutes you could find yourself in heaven.

Imagine, in the middle of your day, you could bring yourself into a state where there is nothing to do, nowhere to go, no one to be and nothing to accomplish. In this place, there is no fear. In this place, you carry no burdens and you feel at peace.

*Paradoxical Relaxation* is the practice of entering into this heavenly kind of sanctuary. This sanctuary isn't exactly how the movies might represent it or how Michelangelo painted it. No feasting rooms, seraphims, trumpets, angels, or pearly gates. There are no buildings, or mountains or streams. In fact there are no forms at all, just a kind of weightless, feathery, light, joyful, effulgent, floating feeling.

> This inner sanctuary is open to everyone
> who has developed the ability to enter it

This heavenly sanctuary is everyone's birthright. It comes with being born. When we see a baby sleeping or happily absorbed in playing with mother, the baby is in this sanctuary. Entrance to it comes to everyone who can rest attention outside of thinking. It can come to us momentarily when we are drifting off to sleep, in a moment of touching someone we deeply love, during a massage, laughing with a child, or listening to beautiful music. This sanctuary is present in everyone all of the time.

This heaven is found in the state of the deepest relaxation. It appears when your thinking stops.

Old mental habits that are deeply ingrained in us from childhood routinely keep us from being able to escape the stresses of the world and calm down inside. For those who want it enough, these old habits can be overcome. With a peculiar kind of devoted practice that I am calling *Paradoxical Relaxation*, it is possible to overcome these habits and deeply relax most any time you want.

Paradoxical Relaxation is the practice of entering into an inner sanctuary

## What typically happens when one becomes profoundly relaxed

When one becomes quiet during *Paradoxical Relaxation*, as in other methods of quieting body and mind, one often experiences a feeling of floating and weightlessness. This is enormously pleasurable and the term ecstasy is not too strong to describe it. Floating is always accompanied by an absence of anxiety. Floating is effortless.

While some who become profoundly relaxed experience floating and weightlessness, others experience a feeling of heaviness, warmth and tingling. People have reported having a sense that they couldn't move, although there was no anxiety connected to this. Sometimes someone who achieves profound relaxation cannot determine if they are lying on their back or their stomach.

It is common during deep relaxation to experience a weight being lifted. As tension reduces, you begin to feel yourself as the agent of protective holding that you did not realize before that you were doing. In the depths of this profound relaxation, there is often a sense of coming home—of returning to a place of such profound comfort that you've always known and is as intimate to you as your breath. At the same time, this most precious experience tends to remain entirely forgotten in the daily course of life.

As one gets into deeper states of relaxation, particularly states that go past the normal range of nervous system quieting with which one is familiar, several unusual kinds of sensations and phenomena can occur. One can experience a kind of jerking and temporary tightening and then relaxation of certain muscle groups at certain stages of *Paradoxical Relaxation*. These are due to a kind of psychophysical ambivalence of letting go of vigilance beyond a certain point. It is as if the body and mind are saying, 'I am letting go now, but as I let go I am not comfortable letting go to the extent I find myself letting go… so I tighten back up to guard against letting go too much, then I let go and go past the point of comfortable letting go and so I tighten up again…."

Sometimes episodic jerking is accompanied by a feeling of falling. The jerking is a defensive response to the sense of falling. At other times deeper levels of relaxation are accompanied by feelings of heaviness of the limbs and a tingling in the arms, hands and feet. Sometimes, momentarily, someone has the feeling that they cannot move (although they always can). Sometimes you have an experience of not knowing whether you are lying on your stomach or lying on your back. Sometimes there's a sense of the body simply disappearing. Again these are all characteristic of deeper states of relaxation.

In systems of yoga, these movements are thought of as involuntary movements, the release of physical, mental, or emotional tension as the life force of *kundalini* moves through areas of tightness. Kriyas are a term in yoga which mean the strong episodic burst of energy.

It is common as parts of the body that have been chronically tightened begin to relax, that one can feel a kind of fluttering or fasciculation in the muscles. It is often pleasant and is usually accompanied by a reduction or cessation of stress related symptoms. Again, this feeling represents a kind of bodily ambivalence of letting go as certain muscles in the body decide whether to relax or tighten.

Some people have followed the relaxation protocol as described in this book and have had some of these experiences and became alarmed by them. In fact, these experiences tend to be good news and are signposts on the road to training the body to come out of its habitual contraction of vigilance and learn to relax.

Becoming competent in *Paradoxical Relaxation* does not occur over night. Over and over again, when you do *Paradoxical Relaxation*, you will confront a multitude of obstacles that interfere with your voluntary ability to relax anxiety and your nervous system. It is in facing these obstacles over and over again that you learn to overcome them.

One way to describe *Paradoxical Relaxation* is to say that it is a practice devoted to entering into the inner sanctuary available to all of us. A more prosaic way of describing the purpose of *Paradoxical Relaxation* is to say that it is a way to stop anxiety, and you get better at it the more you do it.

Anxiety, stress, fear, worry, and agitation, among other terms, are just different names for the same thing. In this book, I use these terms interchangeably. Fear is our response to the perception that our survival in some way is being threatened. As I will describe later, the survival response of fear prompts us to fight, flee, or freeze. The purpose of fear is typically to motivate us to run away from what we feel is threatening. Fear feels bad. None of us like to feel afraid, stressed, or anxious. We all yearn for the feeling of peace and relaxation inside. It has been my experience that in the absence of fear there is the feeling of love, peace, and gratitude. The inner experience of heaven exists in the absence of fear, anger, and emotional agitation.

> Paradoxical Relaxation is a practice devoted to being able to stop anxiety

When you are constantly stressed or anxious, whether or not your body is affected adversely, your nervous system tends to be regularly jacked up and aroused, preventing you from being able to truly rest or relax. Rest and relaxation are the body's medicine to stay healthy and are necessary for the regeneration and recuperation of tissue, and for the maintenance of emotional and physical balance. This inability to deeply relax over time paves the way for *anxiety states* and their related physical difficulties.

## The huge physical, emotional, and existential cost of not being able to relax

The negative effects of prolonged stress are understood throughout our society. Anxiety affects the heart, blood pressure, digestive system, the skin, the immune system, the process of inflammation, the rate of wound healing, among other vital aspects of health. Prolonged anxiety fogs the mind, interferes with sleep, disturbs appetite, and affects sexuality. Even if there were not such a list of negative effects of prolonged anxiety and the inability to relax it, it would be enough reason to learn to relax just to counteract the life and joy-deadening effects of anxiety. When tension and stress is out of our control and we can't calm it down, we pay a huge price. I have both seen the effects of anxiety on the quality of my life and feel great gratitude in having found a way to relax.

## The story you tell yourself about something difficult that happens to you can heal you or cripple you

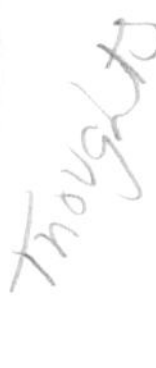

One of the aims of *Paradoxical Relaxation* is to help you to free yourself from your inner stories that keep you agitated and tense. The story you tell yourself when something difficult has happened to you can grant you entrance into your inner sanctuary or lock the door to it. Being able to enter the inner sanctuary of profound relaxation at will is critical, especially in these times.

Richard Gevirtz, David Hubbard, and Ali Oliveira conducted a study on whiplash that is remarkably simple and straightforward in showing the relationship between peoples' physical pain, the utilization of pain medication and medical resources, and their stories of helplessness and catastrophe. These researchers randomly divided up 126 whiplash patients into two well-matched groups. The study group (what we will call the *video group*) was shown a short 12 minute video explaining whiplash as a soft-tissue, reversible injury to the muscles of the neck. This video showed some simple stretching and a simple relaxation method that patients could do to help their symptoms. The video importantly reassured whiplash patients that they could recover. That is all that the *video group* was given. The control group was shown no video (*no-video group*). Both groups were followed up with at one, three, and six months. Simple.

What happened? The results were remarkable. The *no-video group* reported much more pain, much more pain medication use, and much more utilization of medical resources, compared to the *video group.*

Your story about your whiplash injury
can strongly influence its healing

This study demonstrates that giving ordinary people the power to calm down their nervous system, control their catastrophic thinking, and treat their injury with a simple self-help regimen can often spell the difference between being able to recover or not being able to recover from their injury. Conversely *not* reassuring people and *not* giving people the tools to do something for their injury has profound effects. When whiplash patients are not helped in these ways and not helped to dispel any tendency to catastrophize or to feel helpless about their pain, they are at far more risk of being in pain and becoming dependent on pain medication.

## One-third of those who did not see a twelve-minute educational video were using narcotic medications after six months, as opposed to a tiny fraction of those who did see the video

The most remarkable result of this 12 minute video intervention had to do with the fact that at the end of six months, 37% of the *no-video group* was taking narcotic pain medication as opposed to only 2%-4% of the *video group.*

**At six months, compared to the *video* group, the *no-video* group reported:**

- Three times as much pain
- More than seven times the musculoskeletal dysfunction
- Twenty times the number of physical therapy visits
- Seven times the number of MRI's
- Ten times the number of emergency room visits
- Ten times the number of urgent care visits
- Seven times the usage of muscle relaxants
- Ten times the usage of neck braces
- Twenty times the number of surgical consultations
- Five times the number of doctor visits
- Nine times the usage of narcotic medications.

**Nine times the use of narcotic medications after six months in the *no-video* group compared to the *video group***

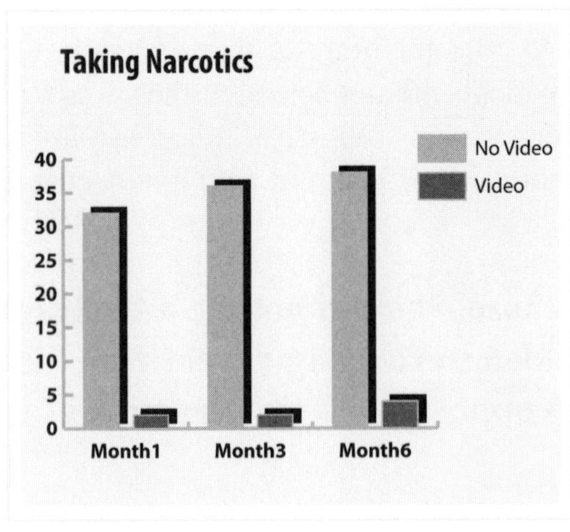

**Other negative consequences of not seeing a 12 minute video after whiplash**

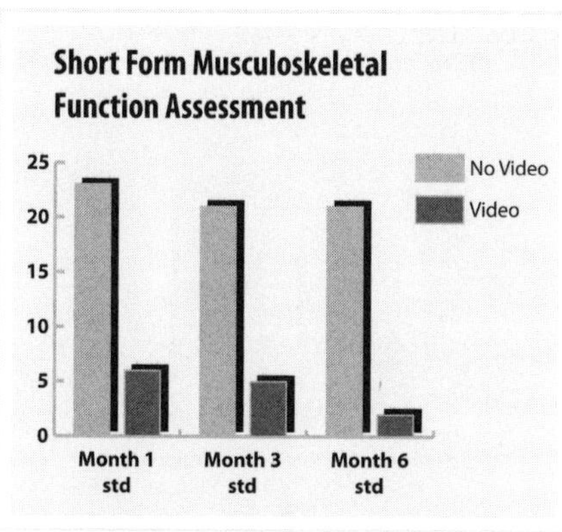


**Disturbance In Function**

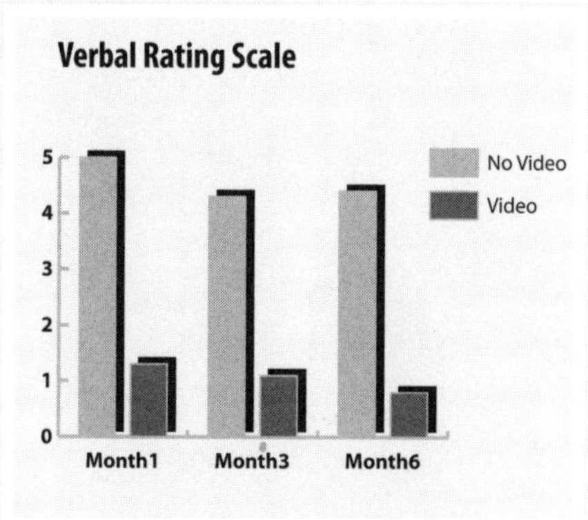


**Pain Rating Scale**

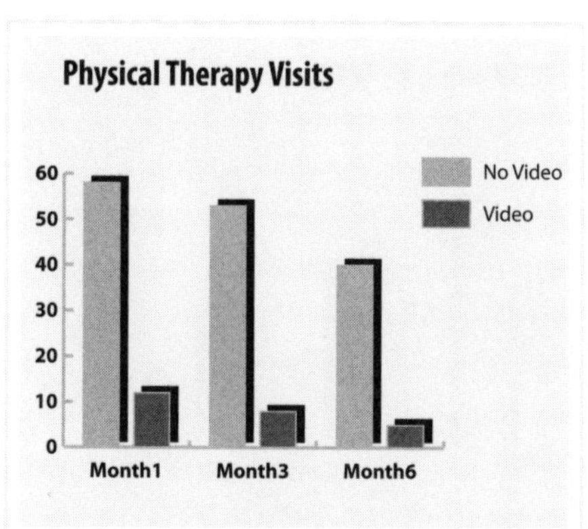


**PT Visits**

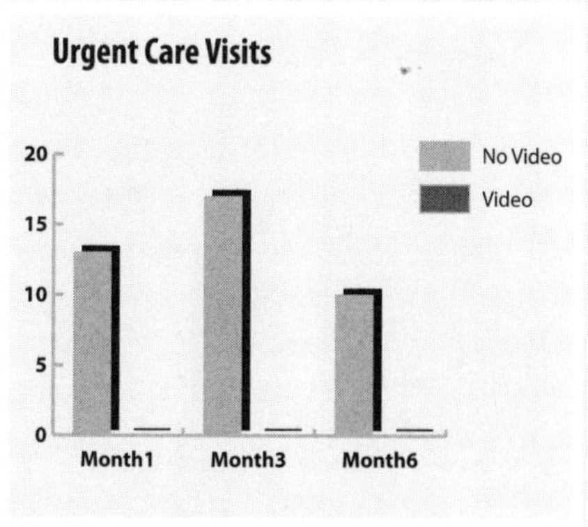


**Urgent Care Visits**

**Other negative consequences of not seeing a 12 minute video after whiplash (continued)**

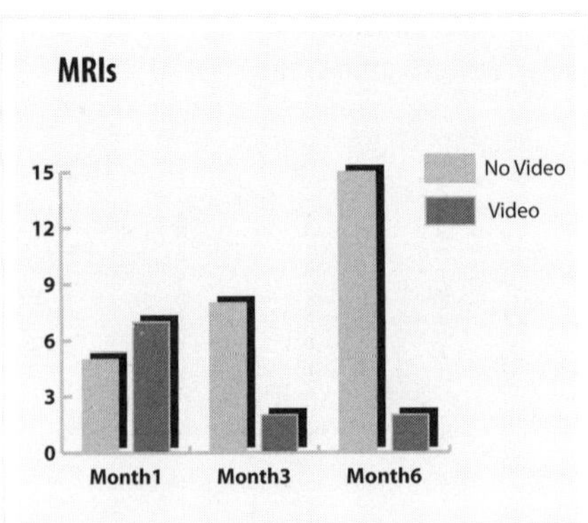


**MRI Usage**



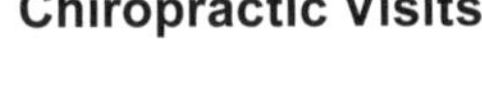

**Chiropractic Visits**

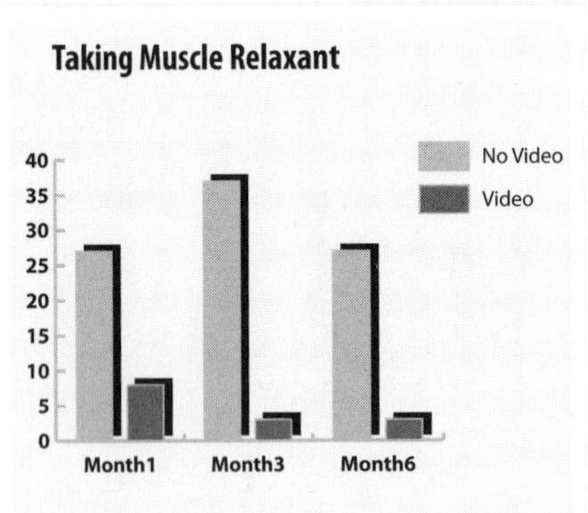


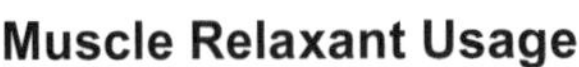

**Muscle Relaxant Usage**

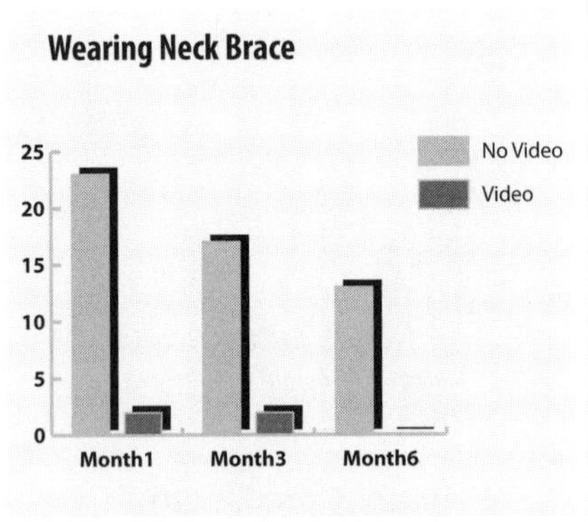


**Use of Neck Brace**

**Other negative consequences of not seeing a 12 minute video after whiplash (continued)**

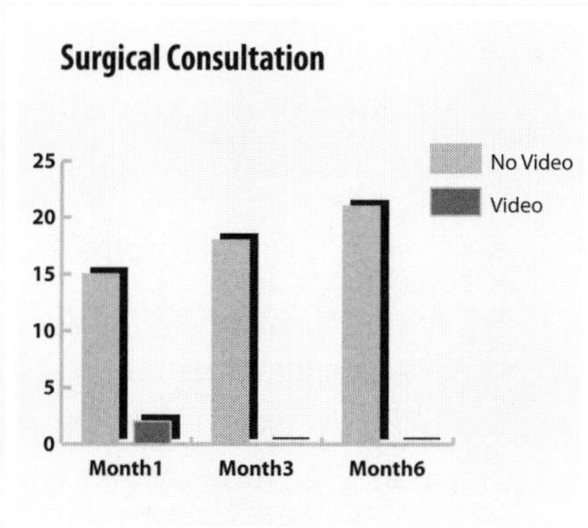


**Surgical Consults**

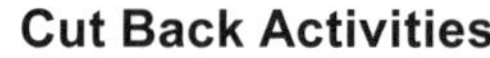


**Cut Back Activities**

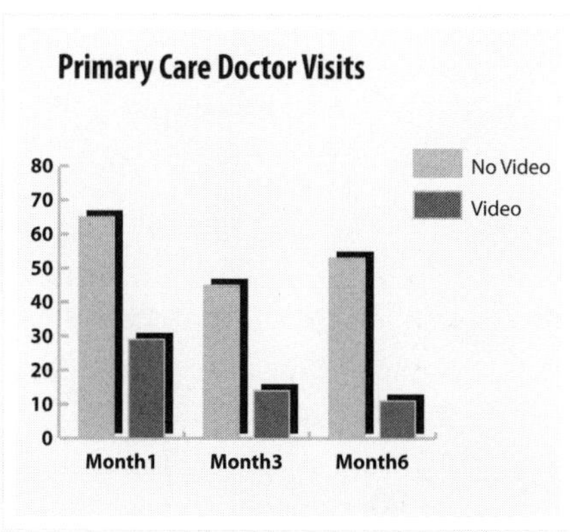


**Primary Care Doctor Visits**

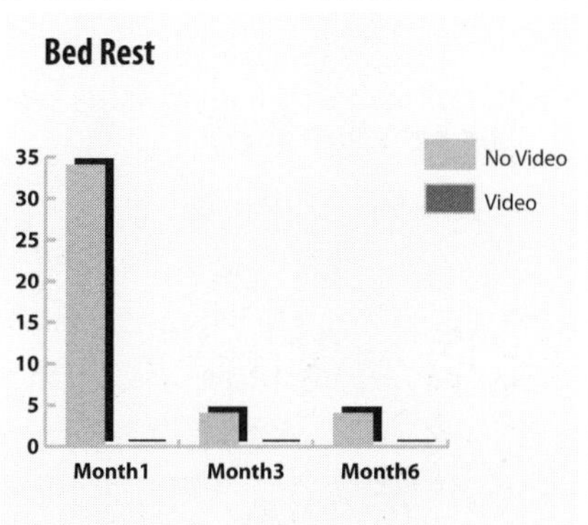


**Bed Rest**

## Why did watching a 12 minute video make such a huge difference in the lives of whiplash victims?

Now the question is, why did watching a 12 minute video produce such results? To answer this, let's examine the intervention. There were three components to the 12 minute video. There was an explanation of whiplash that reassured patients that whiplash was a soft tissue injury that would heal. The video contained instructions on doing a simple breathing/relaxation exercise and some simple stretching to help the healing of the injured neck muscles.

All of these interventions seem innocuous and unlikely to do much. At best the breathing method could have had some limited success in momentarily helping the patient to relax. The stretching technique might have had a small but temporary ability to loosen the tight neck and ease the symptoms. And the video offered an uncomplicated explanation of the nature of whiplash and its ability to heal.

The real power of the 12 minute video, it seems clear, had to do with the overall message that helped people to be unperturbed about their whiplash and its prognosis. The video shaped the way those in the *video group* thought about what was wrong with them after their injury. In reassuring those in the *video group* that everything was going to be alright, and showing them a simple way to help their myofascial pain, the video helped prevent the kind of catastrophic stories and helplessness that often occur in people with whiplash injuries. The video told those who watched it that their whiplash wasn't a bone or nerve problem, with all of the scary implications of bone or nerve injury. In a word, the video helped people relax about their injury and their prospects of recovering from it.

Significantly, those in the study who thought that their injury was a bone or nerve injury had a very high likelihood of having more pain and pain medication use. Why? Because it is easy to catastrophize about a bone or nerve injury and stay in a heightened state of anxiety about it. On the other hand, the video reassured the *video group* that they sustained only a temporary injury to the muscles of the neck and with a little stretching and relaxation, it would heal. It showed them some simple things they could do to calm their nervous system down. With this help, most of them healed easily without incident. Given the innocuousness of the stretching and breathing methods in the video. It gave them a non-catastrophic story about their trauma that helped them to not worry.

> It seems clear that the video ultimately helped most of these whiplash victims not to catastrophize about their injuries. In reassuring them that everything was going to be alright, and showing them a simple way to help their myofascial pain, most of the video group recovered from the injury in a way that many of the no-video group did not

On the other hand, a large percentage of the *no-video group* had significant problems that had the potential to profoundly and negatively affect their entire lives. What appears to have separated those in the *video group* from the *no-video group* was the story they told themselves about what their injury was and what was going to happen to them as the result.

Why I believe this study is so vital is that it shows the effect your story has on your symptoms. The study showed that it is not only neurotic people with troubled childhoods who are prone to a negative inner story affecting their health. It can occur in a large proportion of the population. Ordinary people can affect their health with catastrophic stories. And a medical system that doesn't understand any of this can waste billions of dollars on expensive tests and treatments that do nothing for ordinary people.

When the whiplash patients understood that their whiplash was just reversible pain from muscle as communicated in the video, I believe this understanding resulted in their nervous systems calming down. It resulted in not feeding the mechanisms of tension, anxiety, pain, and protective guarding that perpetuates many kinds of disorders, including whiplash.

And a simple, 12 minute video that helped ordinary people out of their fear and helplessness about their condition, translated into the speedy healing of the whiplash and the avoidance of medical resources that is both costly and of little help. The study strongly points to the fact that what the *no-video* group told themselves about their whiplash prompted the perpetuation and exacerbation of their symptoms. And, for whatever reason, it apparently forced a good one-third of them to turn to narcotic pain medication.

> Learning to calm down your nervous system regularly
> could be more important to your quality of life
> than anything you could ever do for yourself

This study shows the power a chronically upregulated nervous system has on your life and your health. If you suffer an injury or illness and live with a story about your condition that leaves you feeling helpless, this can chronically trigger your nervous system to speed up in preparation for danger. Your muscle-related symptoms will then hurt much more, you may use more medication, and your negative thinking may feed into the cycle that perpetuates your pain. Your story can guide your nervous system to peace or to pain-producing agitation. This study confirms that when your nervous system is aroused too long or too strongly, and you feel no power to control it, all kinds of physical and emotional havoc can result.

When you have a relaxation practice and a way of managing your catastrophic thinking, you don't feed the tension, anxiety, muscle pain and protective guarding cycle that is the central mechanism in many stress-related disorders. It is quite simple. If you don't manage catastrophic thinking and a nervous system that is chronically agitated, the stress-related conditions that you deal with may become chronic.

*Paradoxical Relaxation* is all about regularly bringing yourself back to peace every day. It is about reducing the arousal of your nervous system that has many opportunities during the day to become disturbed. Relaxation and becoming skilled at managing your catastrophic thinking can spell the difference between chronic anxiety, pain and suffering or peace, joy, health, and enjoyment of life.

It is possible to reliably calm down tension, agitation, and anxiety without drugs

In the sped up life of the 21st century, there are many quick fixes available for anxiety. Drugs, alcohol, and other substances are among the most popular. It is no secret that you pay a price for them, especially when you reach for the quick fix regularly.

I have been deeply interested in learning how to relax since I was an anxious young man. From my own experience, I know there is no quick way to learn to calm an agitated nervous system down, especially if you are prone to anxiety or are in pain. If you are looking for a quick method of relaxation, this is not the book for you. There are many CD's and tapes on the internet that offer a quick way to relaxation. In my experience, they typically wind up on the shelf after a few listens. In this regard, I will later discuss the subject and importance of in-person instruction, as opposed to recorded instructions.

The most important requirement in learning to deeply relax is to want it enough. If you want it enough, you can have it

I have practiced and taught *Paradoxical Relaxation* for many years now. In my experience, almost everyone who has truly wanted to experience the fruits of practicing *Paradoxical Relaxation* has been able to do so. In many cases, the ripest students for this practice have said things like, "Enough. There has to be another way. I can't go on like I am," in response to their anxiety and the price their body and mind have paid for it.

There is no royal road in learning to profoundly relax and nobody else can do it for you. Like gaining a pilot's license, you have to simply find the motivation to put in the hours and be sincere about learning the method.

For the first year, *Paradoxical Relaxation* is best done twice, or at least once, every day. Doing the relaxation protocol less than once a day accomplishes little. Arthur Rubenstein, the great pianist, reputedly said that if he missed a day of practice, he noticed it; if he missed two days of practice, his wife noticed it; and if he missed three days of practice, his audience noticed it. For *Paradoxical Relaxation* to work, it must be done every day on an ongoing basis.

The silver lining of the suffering of anxiety is that it can provide the motivation to learn to profoundly relax

The more someone has suffered from anxiety and related difficulties, the more motivated they tend to be to help themselves. You can see this motivation as the silver lining of the suffering. It has the capacity to push you into doing what you would otherwise never do. It is precisely this kind of motivation that can enable someone to persevere through the obstacles of the relaxation protocol in order to learn it. Many patients who were in the most severe kind of pelvic pain when they came to see us for treatment at Stanford, did the best of all of our patients because their level of motivation was the kind that said, "Whatever is necessary to do, I will do."

Most people who learn *Paradoxical Relaxation* do so not because they are looking for heaven, but because they regularly suffer from anxiety, pain, and physical symptoms. I work with many patients who have some physical disorder related to their anxiety and muscle tension. I discuss functional disorders like pelvic pain and irritable bowel syndrome, as well as other conditions, in this book. When these patients learn *Paradoxical Relaxation*, their experience of relaxation typically is accompanied by the reduction and sometimes dissolution of their pain and related symptoms. This is always a good sign and I tell patients to be encouraged by their significant reduction or disappearance of physical symptoms even if at first this is fleeting.

*All of us love to relax.* You can taste food, feel a breeze, imbibe the smell of a rose, and feel your deep caring for others when you are truly relaxed. Chronic anxiety and related disorders always impair our ability to relax. They scuttle the quality of our lives.

I became interested in learning to relax because of my own predisposition toward chronic tension and anxiety. Learning to relax has been and remains a passion for me. It has been a central part of my solution to my tendency to fret, worry, and be tense and anxious. As I look back at my life, I realize I was searching for a way to live without fear from the time I was in my late teens. When I first began practicing *Paradoxical Relaxation,* I would say to myself, "I can relax deeply and easily whenever I want to." I so much wanted to learn to quiet down inside. This affirmation did not magically imbue me with the ability to profoundly relax, but it helped me keep my goal clear. I know that my suffering motivated me to seriously commit myself to learning how to relax. This affirmation was how I cheered myself on.

## ***Suffering as grace*: the suffering of anxiety is what motivates most people to learn how to quiet their anxiety**

Over the last few decades, Ram Dass proposed the idea that suffering can be seen as grace or a gift. *Suffering as grace* means that you come to see that even though you wouldn't choose to have the suffering you are dealing with, nevertheless it turns out to be something precious that may contain the possibility of transforming your life.

Usually the awareness that *suffering is grace* is perceived *after* the suffering has resolved itself. There is a related idea that whatever difficulties you may be facing in a particular moment are not distractions from the curriculum of your life, but are the curriculum itself. Most people believe that their condition has taken their attention away from what they really want to be doing. However, when you look at resolving your anxiety-related difficulties as your *main curriculum,* you bring an entirely different attitude to them. This shift in attitude has the power to transform your difficulties because you stop resisting or hating them. Instead you regard them as your teachers.

There could not be a better use of anyone's time than to learn to live without fear

What does this mean for you if you are suffering from anxiety? Why not view your anxiety as one of the *main courses* that you are enrolled in, in the *university* called your life. In truth, it actually is, whether you like it or not. I am not suggesting in any way that you have deliberately brought anxiety into your life, that you want it there, or that you shouldn't resolve it as soon as possible. I am suggesting the idea that if you do suffer with anxiety, you acknowledge that it is going on and ask yourself the questions: What is my anxiety asking from me? What lesson does my current predicament contain for me? Am I listening?

If you want peace, you have to deserve it by ceasing to do what disturbs your peace

Nisargadatta said that if you want peace, you have to deserve it by not doing what disturbs your peace. What people inwardly do to disturb their inner peace has to do with where their attention is directed. In order to relax profoundly and reliably, you must learn to control your attention. This enables relaxation to occur. Absent the application and practice of these skills, we tend to get batted around by whatever conditioned tendency we have in us that makes us anxious.

Most people are not aware of the many ways in which their thinking and behavior interfere with their inner peace

## ***Paradoxical Relaxation* is 1% inspiration and 99% perspiration**

*Thomas Edison reputedly said that genius is 1% inspiration and 99% perspiration.* The inspiration in *Paradoxical Relaxation* is the instruction and the underlying concepts. The perspiration is the daily, persistent practice of the instructions.

When you are a novice learning relaxation, you often don't appreciate the centrality of one of the main instructions to feel and allow the sensation of tension and anxiety. The novice subtly *tries* to relax even though the instructions given in *Paradoxical Relaxation* urge you to abandon such a strategy.

In *Paradoxical Relaxation,* you are specifically asked *not* to try to relax because you can't try or use effort to deeply relax. After attempting this strategy over and over again, in the face of instructions that specifically ask you *not* to try to relax, the beginner usually comes to see that trying to relax does not work.

It is not uncommon for somebody to do many sessions of relaxation before he or she is earnestly willing to experiment with these instructions—that is to say, when they are willing to genuinely and whole-heartedly feel the tension and anxiety that is present, doing nothing about them.

### Mastering Paradoxical Relaxation requires doing at first what feels like the grunt work of practicing it every day

The moment in which someone is able to feel tension and anxiety and do nothing about them, is a defining moment. It has ramifications and reverberations throughout one's life, as the stage is set for them to experiment with accepting *what is.*

The experience of *Paradoxical Relaxation* is like the experience of Bill Murray in the movie *Groundhog Day.* Each relaxation session is an experience of doing your best to get the practice right, even though it often feels like you have fallen short of the mark, over and over.

There is, however, no way to succeed at *Paradoxical Relaxation* without facing the repeated experience of losing the focus of your attention. The patient must find his or her own way to persevere through these frustrations.

The instructions of *Paradoxical Relaxation* serve to help the patient return to the proper focus and technique, moment by moment. It is easy to get lost in reactions of frustration, doubt, or a sense that nothing is happening. It is the patient's job to notice these reactions, or in other words, *to be a witness to being lost in frustration*, and to re-focus on the instructions without self-rebuke. It is counter-productive for patients to react negatively, however subtly, to straying from the instructions, or becoming lost in thought or frustration. With an attitude of forgiveness and compassion for oneself, the idea is to simply come back into the focus of following the instructions.

In Paradoxical Relaxation we are practicing giving up our holding onto vigilance, defensiveness, self protection, worries, and guarding ourselves

The word surrender comes from the French word *surrendre*, meaning to give up. The practice of *Paradoxical Relaxation* is a practice of letting go of inwardly guarding, bracing, tightening, tensing, squeezing, and contracting. It is a practice of giving up the heavy weight of our daily worries.

**Once you have done everything you are able to do to take care of situations in life that worry you, continued worry is usually a hopeless attempt to control what you cannot control**

The irrational premise of compulsive worrying is that it is not safe for you to take your attention off of what you are afraid might happen. Worry is a certain kind of thinking. Worrisome thoughts focus on the past or future. Worrisome thoughts are the cornerstone of anxiety, stress, and tension. Beyond the positive effect of strongly motivating you to do whatever you need to do about any particular situation, further worry only creates suffering.

When you practice Paradoxical Relaxation and rest attention in sensation beyond the bounds of thinking, you are catapulted into the present moment where worry about the past and future cannot enter

In doing *Paradoxical Relaxation*, you are practicing taking your attention off of all thinking, including worrisome thinking. When you are tense or anxious, your attention is almost always focused in the future or the past. The practice in *Paradoxical Relaxation* of continually bringing attention into the present moment of sensation places you upstream from the anxieties of past and future. When your attention is taken away from worrisome thinking, anxiety and tension connected to worry stops.

The truth is that after you do everything that you can do about any situation, whatever is going to happen is going to happen. In my own life, over and over again, I noticed an inner programming in me that did not allow me to take my attention off of what was worrisome, even when I had no control over it. During a relaxation session, I made and continue to make an existential decision to trust that it is safe for me to take my attention off of worry. This decision, and my ongoing practice has been profoundly important in my ability to calm myself down.

## The mechanics of giving up your burden in the moment during relaxation

When you travel on a train, it makes no sense to carry your luggage on your lap. It makes more sense to let the train carry it. The analogy speaks to the wisdom of surrendering your cares and worries. This is accomplished by withdrawing your attention from worrisome thoughts moment by moment.

Giving up your burden in *Paradoxical Relaxation* requires that you have to *want* to give up your burden. Wanting to give up your burden means being willing to take the risk that it is safe to take your attention off of what is burdening you. Focusing on what is worrisome usually comes from a deeply held idea that paying attention to what is worrisome is necessary to remain safe. I discuss this subject extensively under the heading of pleasure anxiety and the core thought "it is not safe to feel safe." If you are able to inwardly decide to take your attention off of worrisome thinking, and you do so moment to moment in the relaxation session, your muscles relax and your nervous system quiets down. This kind of surrender brings someone to peace. This is the point of *Paradoxical Relaxation.*

## The example of my teachers showed me it was possible to profoundly relax

It was through the examples of all of my teachers that I came to believe that what they taught, in fact, was possible. One of the most important of my teachers was Edmund Jacobson. He was a great source of inspiration for me. It was his example of walking the talk, of being able to deeply relax before my eyes, that inspired me to persevere through my frustration, sense of not knowing what I was doing, and my regular failures at being able to calm down. His example showed me that this kind of relaxation was possible and brought me to this moment in which I can say that my daily relaxation practice is the most precious experience in my life.

There is a proverbial discussion as to whether the stick or the carrot is the best way to motivate someone. In my own case, my own suffering has been the stick in motivating me to relax. The memory of Jacobson's example of profoundly relaxing at will has been the carrot.

## Disturbances of the mind and of the emotions are always disturbances of the physical body as well

When one is chronically anxious, the physical body is unduly taxed. In the younger and stronger person, undue taxation on the nervous system caused by ongoing anxiety may not cause any physical dysfunction or pathology.

However, it takes time for ongoing anxiety to show up in physical symptoms. A younger or hardier person's body tends to be more able to resist the effects of anxiety than an older person's or a less hardy body. Often, with age and an increased duration of anxiety, the body gives in to the nervous onslaught and disturbance of physical functioning can result.

Anxiety-related disorders are *psychosomatic* or *psychophysical* disorders. That is to say, when these states are maintained, they affect *both* the physical and the mental aspects of our organism. Unlike the often dismissive wastebasket category many of these conditions are placed in by frustrated physicians who cannot help them, these conditions are *not* simply mental problems emanating from emotional disturbance. Typically, anxiety affects the body adversely and the body in turn makes the person more anxious. More important, anxiety and anxiety-related disorders are rarely resolved simply by sending someone to a psychiatrist who waves the magic wand of drugs or psychotherapy.

## When anxiety reduces, typically physical symptoms associated with it reduce as well

Regularly calming down disturbance to mind and emotions typically results in the reduction of associated physical symptoms as well. In our work with pelvic pain, it is common to hear that when someone's anxiety reduces, the symptoms of pelvic pain reduce and sometimes stop. When an *anxiety state* resolves, the heart rate, sweat response, blood pressure, increased muscle tension, immune system dampening, and other physical events tend to reduce and come back into balance as well. The body does not say, "I have two components, body and mind." This is a concept imposed on patients by either doctors or conventional thinking that divides mind and body into two separate categories. Particularly in functional disorders, body and mind act as one unit and have no sharp demarcation line to divide them.

I have found that it is more effective to both physically release the parts of the body that have tightened up in anxiety and anxiety-related states *as well as* to practice a method of mental discipline that meaningfully reduces the arousal of the nervous system that inflames the condition. In most cases of people with anxiety, it is necessary for them to regularly stop both the mental and physical habits that tightened up their bodies and caused them distress in the first place.

In the treatment of pelvic pain that we developed at Stanford University, changing the mental *and* physical habits that keep the nervous system aroused and feed anxiety has been the task of the *Wise-Anderson Protocol*. Using *Paradoxical Relaxation* for anxiety with or without associated physical symptoms is the subject of this book.

It is a huge boon to your life to know that
you can stop your own anxiety yourself

In my work with pelvic pain, I have often said that the best anti-anxiety drug is the ability to reduce or stop the anxiety and pain of pelvic pain syndromes *by yourself.* Teaching patients to be able to calm down their own pelvic pain symptoms has become the central purpose of the *Wise-Anderson Protocol.*

One of the essential components of the anti-anxiety strategy I discuss in this book, whether or not you have physical symptoms associated with your anxiety, is to be able to feel a real reduction or absence of anxiety in a half-hour or so relaxation session, without the side effects of drugs.

## The elephant and the blind men and *Paradoxical Relaxation*

*Once upon a time, ten blind men, each with a cane, went for a walk along a road that skirted a jungle. Soon they came upon an elephant, and each one found himself at a different place in relationship to the animal. One blind man touching the elephant's leg remarked, "Oh, this creature is like a tree trunk." Another, who was positioned under the elephant's stomach, pushed up and said, "Oh no. This creature is like a soft ceiling, with nothing else around on the sides." A third positioned at the tail, pulled on it and said, "No, this creature is like a rope connected to a tree." Another, touching the trunk of the elephant, said, "No, this creature is like a large, soft pipe." Yet another, reaching and touching the elephant's tusk, said, "No, this creature is like a curved spear stuck into rock."*

*On and on they argued. What was this creature they had come upon? Finally, a fellow traveler came by and heard the argument. Noticing right away they were blind, he said, "No, you're all correct, and you're all wrong, because this is an elephant and each one of you is only touching one part, thinking that each part constitutes the whole."*

This parable illustrates how something complex can have a number of different sides or aspects that cannot be grasped or described all at once. These different aspects make this object appear different to different people, where they confuse one aspect for the whole thing. When seen with 'unblinded' eyes, these different sides or aspects are shown to all be integral parts of this complex whole.

This parable can be used as a way of understanding the nature of *Paradoxical Relaxation. Paradoxical Relaxation* is like the elephant; it has different aspects that are all necessary components of the whole. One of the aspects has to do with the focus on accepting tension; one has to do with returning attention remorselessly from distraction; one has to do with the intention to continually focus seamlessly without a break in attention. Another aspect has to do with giving up the outcome in favor of staying connected with what the sensation is in the moment or letting go of attachment to feeling better in favor of allowing what is going on to be as it is.

All of these different aspects are really describing one single practice I am calling *Paradoxical Relaxation* aimed at bringing peace to the nervous system. These aspects of the *Paradoxical Relaxation* practice are descriptions, the different components of what is called *Paradoxical Relaxation.* All of the sides or aspects are essential and not one of them alone is sufficient in order to properly practice *Paradoxical Relaxation.*

The order in which these different aspects are done are imperative to the efficacy of the practice. Though it may appear that these aspects are different, separate parts, as you become more skillful at *Paradoxical Relaxation* you begin to intuitively experience the interdependency and intimate relationship between all of these parts to each other. Using another simile, these aspects of *Paradoxical Relaxation* are like the wheels, engine, steering wheel, and exhaust system of a car—all are required to help comfortably and safely move yourself from one place to another. The different aspects of the method I describe work together to allow for the possibility of moving from anxiety to equanimity.

## My personal journey in dealing with my own anxiety

I suffered from a condition called chronic pelvic pain syndrome for many years. For many years, the medical profession was unable to help me, and through my own desire to be free of pain I continued to search out different avenues of treatment. Ultimately I discovered that my pelvic pain was being caused by chronically constricted, tight muscles in and around my pelvis. I further found that this muscle constriction was intimately related to my high levels of anxiety and muscle tension.

Discovering this, I committed myself to a protocol of treatment that combined a certain type of physical therapy with daily *Paradoxical Relaxation* to break my cycle of anxiety, tension, and muscle constriction. Amazingly, this combination of treatment began to help and ultimately freed me from the grips of pelvic pain.

In the gratitude and energy that flowed from my recovery, I began to work with Dr. Rodney Anderson at Stanford University on further developing and refining the protocol, and helping other patients with similar types of pelvic pain. Our treatment was named the *Wise-Anderson Protocol* and Dr. Anderson and I co-authored a book entitled A *Headache in the Pelvis*, which is now going into its 6th edition.

Paradoxical Relaxation was originally used as part of a new treatment for pelvic pain developed at Stanford University

In a nutshell, the *Wise-Anderson Protocol* has two major components. One component focuses on the physical rehabilitation of a chronically contracted pelvic floor. The other component is a mental-behavioral discipline whose purpose is to train patients to relax the pelvic muscles and to reduce the arousal of the patient's nervous system, both key factors in pelvic pain.

Over the years, I tried many methods to calm myself down and stop my pelvic pain. In the methods of relaxation and meditation with which I experimented, I felt unable to release myself from the anxious moods, regular worry, fretting, and often compulsive catastrophic thinking toward which I had a tendency.

Paradoxical Relaxation was a method that emerged in the trenches of closing my own eyes, bringing my attention inside, and dealing with the question of how I could stop the physical pain and anxiety in which I found myself

*Paradoxical Relaxation* came about in my own desperate attempt to stop my chronic pelvic pain and the anxiety that I found myself in. I learned how to do it in the laboratory of my own body, practicing it daily for hours at a time. In this book I only describe what I have experienced. *Nothing that I say here is simply theoretical.* I have endeavored to only share what has been tested in the laboratory of my own relaxation practice.

I found that tension relaxed when I accepted it and not when I tried to get rid of it

*I discovered in my own body over and over again that I had to give up trying to relax in order to profoundly relax. Trying* to relax never worked. What that means is that in order to for me to profoundly relax, I paradoxically had to give up wanting my experience in a particular moment to be any different from the way it actually was. I had to give up trying to relax in order to relax. Understanding this and experiencing this deeply was a changing point in my life and this insight is the subject of this book.

I found there were many barriers to me even noticing my feeling of resistance to the experience in my body. In fact, I found numerous very subtle but stubborn resistances inside me; resistances to simply feeling uncomfortable sensations in my body. When I finally got it—that there was no point in going to war against these resistances as I had fruitlessly done for many years—my inner life changed and my ability to relax profoundly deepened.

My exploration of how to relax occurred silently within myself. Learning to quiet down inside is a profoundly solitary experience. You do it alone. Few people share this aspiration and fewer I have met have devoted real time and energy to exploring how to do it. Fewer have any *real* ability to do it.

*Paradoxical Relaxation* has been a fierce method for me. It has required and continues to require me to face the gamut of my inner experience, from the scary to the sublime. I have come to see that if I am really serious about quieting myself down deeply, I have to allow every subtle expression of fear, anxiety, sorrow, sadness, aversion, dislike, and boredom, among other unpleasant emotions that arise in me. I have come to see that *learning to relax means fully accepting my inner experience.* I discovered that facing these feelings means primarily feeling them in the moment as physical/emotional sensations in my body.

The main struggle of everyone learning Paradoxical Relaxation is remaining undaunted and undisturbed in the face of what at first feels like an incorrigibly wandering and distracted mind

The first challenge is managing your reaction to not being able to focus. I struggled with learning to focus my attention for years without understanding that controlling my attention was one of the main requirements in being able to profoundly relax.

Throughout my life, I was aware of how my attention would jump from one thing to the next and how often I would get lost in the movies of my mind. I remember once as a young man in my 20's, doing renovation in the kitchen of a house I had bought and noticing that I felt miserable while doing it because my mind was jumping from one unpleasant thought to the next. I knew I was doing this mental jumping around, but had no idea what to do about it or that anything could be done about it. I didn't even have a name for my attention being so out of control. My attention was out of my control throughout most of my life.

# Chapter 2

## Overview of *Paradoxical Relaxation*

## ***Paradoxical Relaxation* is a method consisting of a set of instructions about what to do with you attention in order to profoundly relax**

*Paradoxical Relaxation* is not a pill or a scalpel or a splint. It is not a physical object. *Paradoxical Relaxation is a set of instructions that guide your attention during a 25-45 minute relaxation session.* I recommend that these sessions are done once or twice a day on an ongoing basis.

In this chapter, I will discuss the nuts and bolts of *Paradoxical Relaxation.* I will discuss its theory and practice in influencing the subtle adjustment in your attention toward your inner experience during relaxation. Instructions on how to subtly adjust your attention toward your inner experience can at first sound strange and perplexing if you are unaccustomed to bringing attention inside yourself.

That *Paradoxical Relaxation* is a set of instructions about what to do with your attention, for many people, will make it appear to be a very peculiar form of healing. For some, a set of instructions about what to do with your attention can appear to have no substance, no teeth, no power, no ability to heal, or do anything of any value. Upon reading this book I can imagine someone's inner skeptic saying, "What is this guy talking about? How is this kind of stuff going to do anything?"

Regular, profound relaxation can do
what no drug or surgery can do

Training the body to deeply relax in the way I describe in this book can do what no drug and no surgery can do. It can be one of the keys to living a life free from debilitating anxiety, resolving certain conditions of crippling pain, and healing certain conditions that afflict the body. And it can do this by specifically training attention to focus inside the body for regular periods of time. If you have little experience with relaxation training or meditation, some of the discussion of the subtleties of holding attention may at first be obscure and difficult to understand.

For those who have experience in relaxation training or meditation, or who are willing to be open to what I discuss below, as is the case with most of my patients, the information in this book will be of great interest and help.

Paradoxical Relaxation is the practice of conscious effortlessness

*Paradoxical Relaxation* is a practice of ceasing effort by accepting tension and resting attention in sensation. It is a practice of conscious effortlessness. Conscious effortlessness means you are awake and present and exerting not an iota of effort. I have been careful to use language that I believe best communicates the paradoxical insights that allow the body to come into a state of peaceful repose.

## *Paradoxical Relaxation* gets real about the real-life obstacles to lying down and doing a relaxation session

*Paradoxical Relaxation* addresses the real-life, moment to moment inner obstacles to relaxation. *Paradoxical Relaxation* is designed to help someone who is anxious or in pain manage the often overwhelming distraction of anxiety or pain in order to enter into a state of conscious effortlessness. The instructions of *Paradoxical Relaxation get real* about helping someone who is suffering with anxiety or anxiety-related symptoms to lie down and calm down the nervous system.

It takes courage to do Paradoxical Relaxation. To profoundly relax, you are asked to lie down, stay awake, rest your attention in sensation and allow anxiety or discomfort to come and go in your awareness without doing anything to change them

When you are anxious or in pain, it is difficult and almost always scary and unpleasant at first to lie down to do a relaxation session because it means being alone with anxiety, discomfort, and uncertainty. The aversion to these feelings and what to do with that aversion scuttles the attempt of many to put an end to their anxious state using their own efforts.

The instructions of *Paradoxical Relaxation* specifically address what to do with the subtle psychological resistances to lying down with anxiety and discomfort. They address the issue of attention and how central it is to commit yourself to developing the muscle of attention. The instructions of *Paradoxical Relaxation* directly focus on going beyond the reflex to avoid pain and move toward pleasure in the relaxation session itself.

When you are motivated to learn relaxation, you are often upset emotionally in some way. These emotions are usually unexpressed and remain inside and are felt as a certain kind of pressure, constriction, or deadness and, when unresolved, are obstacles to your nervous system calming down. Noticing these emotions during relaxation is essential. Fear, sadness, grief, anger, frustration are among the kinds of emotions that can be present during relaxation. What do you do if they arise during relaxation? The instructions of *Paradoxical Relaxation* directly address what to do with these emotions when they arise.

Anxiety and chronic tension are states of self-defense. When you are anxious or chronically tense, there is some deep part of you, usually unspoken and unconscious, that feels like you have to protect yourself. In a kind of unconscious reasoning, some part of your mind believes that tension and anxiety are helping you stay safe. I discuss this later as pleasure anxiety, catastrophic thinking, and the desire to avoid disappointment by rejecting the experience of feeling safe.

Pleasure anxiety and the fear of feeling safe and undefended are not just concepts. They occur in real people who are suffering. Pleasure anxiety and the fear of feeling safe remain obstacles to relaxation if they are not addressed directly with the aim of overcoming their influence.

## *Paradoxical Relaxation* is the practice of undefending yourself

If tension is part of your way of defending yourself, *Paradoxical Relaxation* is the practice of letting go of defending yourself. When people who are anxious or suffering from the symptoms of anxiety come in to learn *Paradoxical Relaxation,* they usually feel fear about letting go. Sometimes people are apprehensive about what they will find inside, or nervous that they may lose control, or that something bad will happen if they let down. The premise, which I make explicit in *Paradoxical Relaxation*, is that the natural state, under all the agitation of the nervous system, is one of peace. This is a fundamental understanding in wisdom traditions throughout history.

## Underneath anxiety is peace

I tell patients that they only have to trust the instructions of *Paradoxical Relaxation* up to the point where they have their own experience of the ultimate safety of resting in the state of deep relaxation. It is important to specifically say to people, "Underneath all of your suffering, your tension, anxiety and pain, is peace and equanimity. You only have to trust my words until you have the experience of this yourself. Then it is your experience and you don't have to rely on what I say anymore. In other words, it is safe to rest with anxiety, fear, sorrow, doubt, and uncertainty because underneath all of these disturbing emotions is what you are looking for." If you don't talk about the anxiety, fear, sorrow, doubt, and uncertainty, and address them in relaxation instructions, it is my experience that they can remain huge obstacles.

In *Paradoxical Relaxation*, the foundation of treatment is the basic premise that relaxation occurs in the presence of mental quiet. I tell patients that anxiety is a disturbance of their natural state of peace and equanimity. The capacity for resting in a state without fear is never gone. Mental and emotional disturbance obscure the natural anxiety-free state of inner quiet.

To become skilled in *Paradoxical Relaxation* it is necessary to be committed to daily practice. Without real earnestness, reliable and ongoing ability to relax is not possible. *Paradoxical Relaxation* instructions exhort the student to stay committed to following the instructions on a moment to moment basis.

*Paradoxical Relaxation* is best done in conjunction with cognitive therapy and physical stretching of parts of the body that are chronically tightened. This combination is in the great tradition of systems of yoga and meditation that have passed the centuries-old test of time.

## Limitations of conventional methods of relaxation

The treatment of anxiety using relaxation training has been the step-child of conventional psychology . It has been the janitor in the hierarchy of psychiatric interventions. In recent years, medications have been at the top of the hierarchy. A friend of mine has a son who is having a difficult time during his first semester at college. When he went in to the school counseling center for some help, two different psychotherapists suggested drugs during the first 15 minutes of the first interview. I have observed that many psychotherapists, whom I believe are concerned about peer evaluation of their treatment and malpractice, routinely refer patients for medication. In my mind, the message is, "If you are troubled or anxious, even if you are doing psychotherapy, it may be good to take drugs as well." I myself have grown up with the idea that drugs should be used for dealing with mental and emotional difficulty only when absolutely necessary. I don't agree with a policy of giving drugs easily or automatically as a first treatment for depression, anxiety, or other emotional difficulties.

Little serious controlled research and associated funding have been devoted to relaxation methods. There is little money to be made from these methods and even government funds not aimed at profit have been scarce in supporting this kind of research in comparison to drug research.

In addition, research studying relaxation methods have typically been the least respected of studies, because they have often been underfunded, uncontrolled and performed by non-medical practitioners who, again, had little research funding. If psychiatrists or psychologists teach relaxation, their training tends to be minimal. It is not a hot subject in medical schools. Relaxation training is rarely the focus of therapy for anxiety and is at best considered an adjunct to it.

Relaxation therapy tends to be referred to in the same breath as exercise or eating well. In the scientific literature, research on the efficacy of relaxation for different conditions typically involves studies lasting twelve weeks or less. I know that this is a woefully inadequate time period for study subjects to achieve competence in any relaxation method.

Relaxation training tends to be something that is discussed at the end of a session for anxiety in a variety of therapies. The therapist may give the patient a tape or CD with the instructions to go home and use it. The assumption is that listening to someone encouraging you to relax can offer you a way to turn down a chronically aroused nervous system in the midst of anxiety, catastrophic thinking, and the discomfort of pain or physical symptoms related to anxiety.

In mainstream relaxation training, the psychological resistances to becoming quiet inside tend not to be addressed. Pleasure anxiety and the common core thought that, 'It is not safe to feel safe,' to my knowledge are rarely discussed or dealt with. Long-term instruction and follow up are rare. The requirement of training attention to stay focused is rarely considered. Instruction about remorse over losing focus or not being able to satisfy inner expectations about being able to relax are rarely addressed. Often patients are trained in visualization without addressing the effects of eye movement on relaxation, effects that can be significant as eye movement during relaxation interferes with achieving the deepest level of relaxation.

## How *Paradoxical Relaxation* training is outside of the box of conventional relaxation training

Instead of avoiding addressing what is disturbing, not relaxing, or uncomfortable, *Paradoxical Relaxation* instruction regularly and necessarily focuses on what to do with unrelaxing cognitions and thoughts. In the didactic discussion of the principles that underlie a formal relaxation session, *Paradoxical Relaxation* encourages patients to identify often unconscious core thoughts, usually conditioned in childhood, that resist complying with the relaxation method's instructions and release them.

In *Paradoxical Relaxation,* the premise is that the relaxed state occurs when mental activity is quiet. The most restful sleep is non-REM sleep where there are no dreams or mental activity. The reduction of mental activity is the requirement for the most profound and rejuvenative relaxation. I sometimes call *Paradoxical Relaxation* non-REM *Relaxation.*

## *Paradoxical Relaxation* is based on principles that have been used over the centuries to calm down body and mind

Tested in the laboratory of my own practice over the years, *Paradoxical Relaxation* borrows from what I believe are the universal principles that, when skillfully practiced, quiet down body and mind. *These principles have existed for time immemorial. I did not invent these principles. No one owns them. All effective meditation and relaxation practices borrow from them. I have simply borrowed the principles that, in my experience, specifically addressed how to relax in the presence of anxiety, muscle tension, and related physical symptoms.*

## Accepting stubborn tension is the sword that cuts the Gordian Knot of stubborn tension

Normally when you feel tension in the body and you give yourself the instruction to relax it, the nervous system responds by following your instruction. Chronic tension associated with anxiety has a mixed response to this kind of instruction. I struggled for many years to no avail, with the question of how to relax my chronic tension and the anxiety related to it.

What I have found that brings stillness to the body and mind is not new. It has been known to adepts of meditation systems throughout the ages, but the discovery of it was new to me. One of my discoveries involved the unlikely observation that resting with and accepting tension relaxes it.

There is an ancient myth about Alexander the Great and the Gordian Knot. A prophecy existed that anyone who could undo an intricately tied knot would become the king of Asia. Many men tried unsuccessfully to untie the knot. Myth has it that Alexander approached the knot, withdrew his sword, and cut the knot in half. This story has been used over the centuries to illustrate a solution that solved a problem that had perennially defied solution. The *acceptance* of tension, anxiety, and pain in the practice of *Paradoxical Relaxation* is the sword that cuts the Gordian Knot of tension, anxiety, and pain.

In the relaxation session, you can most easily dissolve what is unpleasant by turning toward it and doing nothing about it

Dissolving tension by accepting it equally applies to the dissolution of all that tends to be unpleasant in states of anxiety. In *Paradoxical Relaxation,* we directly and deliberately talk about anxiety and what is unpleasant and uncomfortable, both before initiating relaxation as well as in the actual instructions during relaxation. I ask patients to look at their automatic attitude towards their anxiety and pain and notice any fear they might have about their pain and anxiety. I ask them to notice their natural reactions of flight or avoidance. I encourage patients to stop regarding these sensations as enemies or as experiences to avoid.

This has to be practiced over and over again to get good at it. The result of doing this consistently continues to amaze me.

## Symptom threshold: proximity to the threshold determines how much stress you can handle until you trigger anxiety or related symptoms

To some degree or another, anxiety is just part of everyone's life. No one would suggest you can eliminate anxiety entirely. Imagine a threshold on a graph measuring anxiety and nervous system arousal. When the arousal of the nervous system goes above the threshold, anxiety occurs, when it falls below, anxiety ceases.

In *Paradoxical Relaxation,* what we want to do is bring the baseline level of nervous arousal to a point well below the threshold. When the nervous system activity is well below the symptoms threshold, stress can raise the nervous system arousal without crossing over the threshold. Another person who, in one moment is not anxious, becomes anxious with little provocation, the activity of their nervous system usually rests right below the symptom threshold (positions *E* and *F* in Figure 1). When someone is anxious much of the time but occasionally stops being anxious, their usual position of nervous system arousal on the arousal graph is slightly above the symptom threshold (*C* and *D* in Figure 1).

When someone's nervous arousal is substantially below the symptom threshold, they almost never get anxious as their nervous system arousal rarely goes above the symptom threshold (position *H* in Figure 1). When someone is well below the symptom threshold, even difficult and large amounts of stress don't trigger anxiety. When someone is near the symptom threshold (positions *E* and *F* in Figure 1), apparently insignificant things like someone not smiling at you or someone calling but not leaving a message can trigger anxiety.

Figure 1
Graph of nervous system arousal

| | |
|---|---|
| | A |
| High nervous system arousal (high anxiety and related symptoms) | B |
| | C |
| (above threshhold) | D |
| SYMPTOM THRESHOLD | |
| (below threshold) | E |
| | F |
| Low nervous system arousal (no anxiety or related symptoms) | G |
| | H |

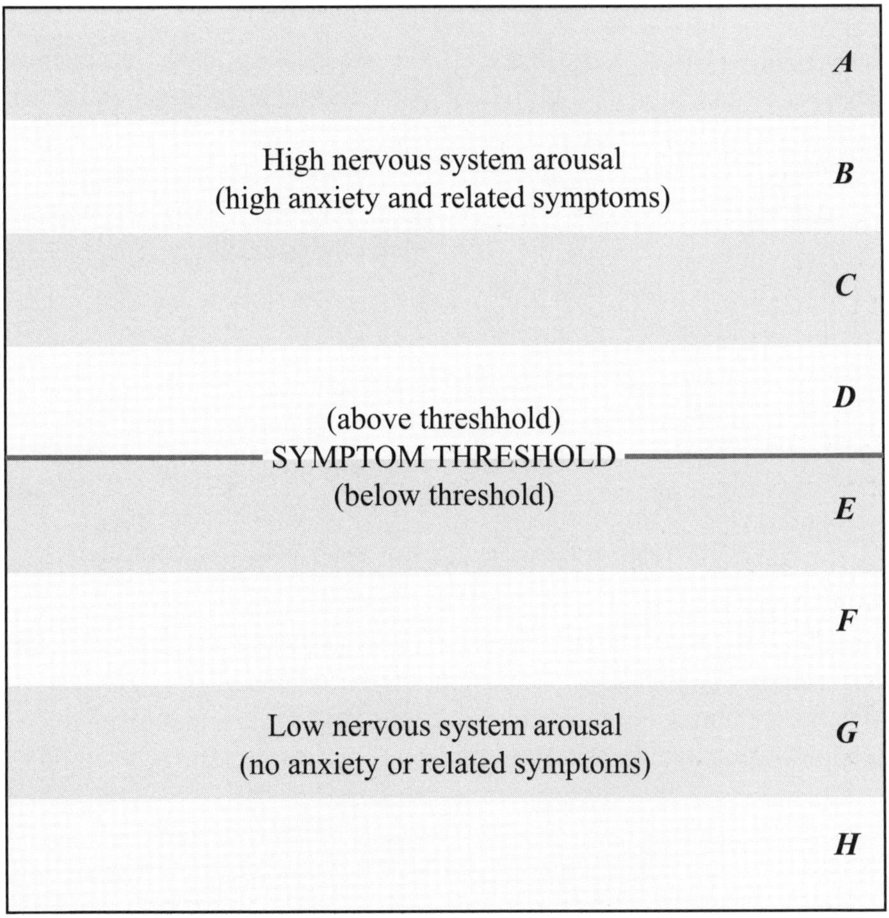

## The nervous systems of fear and relaxation: the sympathetic and parasympathetic divisions of the autonomic nervous system

Let me begin by talking about the autonomic nervous system involved in both the experience and the absence of stress. This autonomic nervous system has two branches, called the sympathetic and the parasympathetic branches, which regulate what have traditionally been thought of to be involuntary functions of the body, like the functioning of the heart, lungs, blood pressure, temperature, and pupil size, bowel and sexual organs, glands and blood vessels, among many other structures.

I want to give a simplified version of the physiology of stress in context with *Paradoxical Relaxation.*

This book describes a method that puts the arousal of your autonomic nervous system under a degree of your control that is generally not thought possible by conventional models of the nervous system. Recent advances in neuroscience and studies in nervous system self-regulation have changed the idea of a solely involuntary autonomic nervous system, as autonomic functioning can very much be positively influenced by certain kinds of behavioral practices.

> You can think of the two branches of the autonomic nervous system as consisting of red and green wires: the red wires, among other functions, can conduct warning signals to the body, the green wires send 'all is okay' signals

These two branches of the autonomic nervous system can be visualized as consisting of either red wires or green wires. I'll call the sympathetic nervous system the red wires. Under certain circumstances in which you perceive a threat of some kind, your sympathetic nervous system is flooded with nervous impulses. In the common vernacular, when someone is 'jacked up,' their sympathetic nervous system is buzzing with activity. The person might be sweaty, nervous, jumpy, reactive at a hair trigger, and panicky.

Sympathetic arousal is by no means always bad. The sympathetic nervous system is the nervous system of activity and is aroused when you are excited, enthusiastic, or energetic. Anxiety is simply a certain kind of sympathetic nervous system arousal. It is *chronic* arousal that is the problem.

Let's think of the green wires of the parasympathetic nervous system as the cool down, 'chill out,' calming down nervous system. Think of it as sending cool, relaxing pulses to the different structures in the body, that say to them, "Everything is cool, everything is okay, relax."

The sympathetic branch of the nervous system has traditionally been thought to manage the organism's arousal, the fight, flight, freeze reaction that enables the organism to survive in an environment which threatens its survival. The parasympathetic division of the nervous system has to do with the organism's regeneration of itself, the repairing of tissue, the managing of the things in the body that need to be managed for the health and comfort of the organism.

When there is a fire in your apartment,
you postpone doing the laundry

Think about all of the routine, daily tasks you do in your life. Tasks like cleaning your apartment, paying your bills, buying and preparing food, doing the laundry. It goes without saying that if there's a fire in the apartment building, you postpone vacuuming your floor or making a shopping list. Your response to the fire in the apartment building causes you to postpone the things you normally do to take care of your life in order to survive. Once the fire is put out, you can go back to the routine tasks that can be done at your leisure.

When I talk about someone being 'sympathetically aroused' I am saying the part of the nervous system with the red wires is stimulating the organism to protect itself because of some kind of signal, realistic or not, that its survival is threatened. Adrenaline is secreted, heart rate and blood pressure increase, muscles tense, blood sugar levels rise, energy increases, pupils dilate and sweating occurs. Functions that are not essential to immediate survival, transmitted by the green wires, including digestion, sexual arousal, immune response and white cell production are reduced. These kinds of activities and functions are meant to be reduced on a short term basis, like putting out the fire before doing the laundry.

We would never decide permanently to stop doing the laundry, stop cleaning our apartment, stop showering, or stop paying our bills because we once had a fire. Sympathetic arousal is not meant to be chronic or ongoing. But if we had an ongoing fire, it would be hard to do normal housekeeping tasks in our life. The problem is when nervous system activity is chronically turned up over time as in *anxiety states*. When these states go on for too long and are on too strongly, they cause certain parts of the body to stop working properly. When the stress is chronic, pathological changes in structure as well as function can occur.

The green wires of the parasympathetic nervous system act in an opposite way to the sympathetic activity, giving the body room to recuperate and regenerate. Parasympathetic nervous system arousal promotes muscles to relax, breathing to slow down and deepen, digestion and peristalsis (rhythmic and healthy movement) of the bowel and the esophagus to resume, stomach digestive fluids to resume normal activity, and so on.

The parasympathetic nervous system is the nervous system of relaxation, pleasure, deep sleep, rest, enjoyment, recuperation, joy, love and peace. It has been thought that when the sympathetic system is activated, the parasympathetic system is reciprocally reduced and when the parasympathetic system dominates, the sympathetic system is inhibited.

## The *up-regulated nervous system*

The term *up-regulated nervous system* has come into use to describe a chronically aroused nervous system operating too fast and at too high an *idle speed.* The *up-regulated nervous system* is like the engine of a car whose owner is pressing down on the gas pedal while in neutral. When the car engine's speed is going too fast for too long a time, the different parts of the car, like the tires, drive shaft, fuel system, car displays, and brakes—can be stressed to the point of failure.

Words that describe an *up-regulated nervous system* are: nervous, jumpy, anxious, uptight, worried, scared, freaked, in an *anxiety state*, sympathetically aroused, panicked. Words that describe a *down-regulated nervous system* are: relaxed, chilled out, cooled down, peaceful, tranquil, happy, harmonious, cool, calm.

Paradoxical Relaxation allows you to regularly turn down your idle speed and lower your baseline level of anxiety

Using the car engine analogy, the purpose of *Paradoxical Relaxation* is to allow you to open up the hood, get into the engine, and properly adjust the lever regulating how hard the engine is working. In adjusting this lever, the engine can slow down to a normal speed that does not stress the car engine or parts of the car that it runs.

When Walter Canon opened up the abdomen of a cat, it's bowel moved rhythmically when the cat was undisturbed but stopped moving when a dog was brought into the room

In Walter Canon's experiments at Harvard during the first part of the 20th century, he opened up the abdomen of a cat and noticed that the cat's bowel moved rhythmically and regularly. When a dog was brought in the room, the peristaltic movement of the bowel stopped. In the first case, the cat was in a parasympathetic mode of nervous system arousal. Enter the dog and the parasympathetic nervous system immediately was inhibited as the sympathetic nervous system took over. When the dog was taken out of the room, the bowel of the cat resumed its peristalsis. Sympathetic dominance (increased activity in the red wires) momentarily occurred and then subsided at which time parasympathetic dominance prevailed (predominance of green wire signals).

Relaxing muscle tension can break the chain of events that keeps anxiety going

When we feel our survival is threatened in some way, our nervous system mobilizes to meet the threat. This mobilization is a biological necessity for any species to survive. Walter Canon's typology of "fight, flight, and freeze," no matter which component of the survival response is called into action, requires muscle contraction. Along with other characteristic physiological responses to a threat, muscle contraction is a necessary event in surviving on earth.

When an organism survives a threat and is home free, unnecessary muscle contraction releases. Muscle tension used for fight, flight or freeze is no longer needed. The problem in certain functional disorders occurs when the muscles have been held tight much longer and more strongly than they are meant to remain contracted.

## *Paradoxical Relaxation* is aimed at reducing arousal of a nervous system stuck on the "on" position

When any of these systems, including the system of muscles, are called upon to be in an emergency mode for too long, they sometimes get stuck in the 'on' position. This is especially problematic when it occurs in the early formative years when the organism is vulnerable, like in the case of parental abandonment or abuse, and the subconscious 'remembers' these emergency states and perpetuates them later in life. In these cases, even though the original trigger for the emergency is long past it can somehow be elicited again by events later in life that call upon this unresolved emergency state. This ongoing perpetuation of the emergency reaction occurs when tension, anxiety, pain, and protective guarding feed each other and tend to take on a life of their own.

Erik Erikson in *Childhood and Society* said that the first stage in life is a stage in which the child inwardly feels a sense of safety or non-safety. He called this stage *trust versus mistrust.* I suggest there are at least three important factors contributing to the foundation of our inward sense of safety. One is a natural physical predisposition toward inward balance or fretfulness. We all know that a fretful baby can appear like it comes out of the womb fretful, even in the most loving of families. This factor refers more to the heredity side of the heredity-environment continuum in what influences personality styles.

Then there are the environmental factors, of which I would like to briefly discuss two important components. They are the factors of how you were treated as an infant and young child and what degree of safety your parents felt in their own worlds.

## Loneliness, anxiety, and *Paradoxical Relaxation*

Loneliness and anxiety are kissing cousins. In the extreme, when human beings experience loneliness, they hold the thought that in some sense they are cast out of human society, that they are exiled from the care, protection, and love of others. You look at the village from a distance, but are not part of it. The human being is a social animal having existed perennially in groups. Thoughts that the love, care and protection of the group is not available to you can trigger anxiety about survival itself. This is why anxiety and loneliness usually exist together.

My main point in this discussion of loneliness is that *loneliness like anxiety, is an inner experience of contraction* and is ultimately not about outer circumstances. *This inner contraction is triggered and perpetuated by a thought.* Loneliness comes from a thought. When focus on the thought goes away, so does loneliness. In a moment, a few words like, "I love you" or, "Come to dinner" can sometimes temporarily make loneliness disappear as the thought that you are all alone and unloved disappears.

When you are skillful at Paradoxical Relaxation, it is possible to relax the inner contraction of loneliness when it arises

Being able to release yourself from the thought-feeling of loneliness can be a life changing experience. As with any deep, habitual, self-protective state, dealing with loneliness is never resolved forever in one moment. It is dealt with daily during each particular episode of the experience of loneliness. Using *Paradoxical Relaxation* in working with loneliness, you repetitively relax *with* the contraction of loneliness, and practice releasing yourself from the loneliness-generating thoughts that keep your heart closed and your spirit small.

> *"Our language has wisely sensed the two sides of being alone. It has created the word loneliness to express the pain of being alone. And it has created the word solitude to express the glory of being alone."*
>
> *Paul Tillich*

Even though there are circumstances in which you can be lonely in a crowd or in your own family, loneliness and solitude have the common outer experience of there being no intimate person present in the moment. Loneliness and solitude are, however, universes apart in their respective inner experiences. Loneliness, as I define the experience, almost always feels bad. Solitude, as I define the experience, almost always feels good.

In loneliness, in the extreme, you hold the thought that, "I am separate and alone, I am locked out of the house of love, connection, joy, and peace. No one is here for me. No one will take care of me if I need care. No one loves me." When someone holds the loneliness-generating thought, their body almost always self-protectively contracts.

In solitude, you *do not* hold the thought that you are exiled from love and care even though no one is immediately around. In the state of solitude, with no thoughts that trigger fear, you experience your own natural state of peace, wholeness, gratitude and love. Even if no one is there, you feel related to humanity. The body of someone who experiences solitude tends to be one of ease, relaxation, pleasure, and enjoyment in being alone. Here again, the difference between loneliness and solitude is an inner state triggered (or not triggered) by a thought and not an outside circumstance.

The misunderstanding that loneliness is about your outer circumstances—the result of living alone without an intimate other or not being in a romantic or family relationship—keeps many people living lives of quiet desperation. They think that they need a loving or intimate person present to feel okay and if that person isn't there, so the misunderstanding goes, there is no answer to their loneliness. The internet dating sites are populated by many people who share this misunderstanding.

*"When people are lonely they stoop to any companionship."*

*Lew Wallace*

Of course, it is sometimes possible to resolve loneliness by being in association with others, as being with others can remove the loneliness-generating thought that you are beyond care and love. People who have supportive social networks, in general, live longer and are healthier. Indeed sometimes 'meeting someone,' can stop the experience of loneliness. *Going to the Chapel*, the popular 1950's song by the Dixie Cups, is a celebration of the hope that someone else can cure your loneliness. The lyrics are:

*Spring is here, the-e-e sky is blue,*
*whoa-oh-oh, birds will sing as if they knew,*
*Today's the day, we'll say I do*
*And we'll never be lonely anymore*

However, 'meeting someone,' as we all know, does not guarantee that loneliness is banished. Stories of the failure of relationships to cure loneliness are legion. We see everywhere the failure of the myth that romantic relationship protects you from loneliness. The marriage counseling industry is a testimony to this.

The same principle that others don't necessarily cure loneliness applies to non-romantic relationships like family and friends. Certainly a loving and supportive family can be of great comfort. I have seen individuals in psychotherapy, however, who have lived apart from their large families for years, have moved long distances to be with their families again because they felt lonely, and to their disappointment and dismay, found that their inner state of loneliness and isolation didn't go away. Similarly, I have seen many individuals who felt a great disappointment that their children ultimately didn't cure their deep feeling of isolation and being unloved as they had hoped. Their children grew up and started their own lives and the inner lives of their parents remained the same as before their children came on the scene.

The common experience of loneliness is usually the experience of isolation. It tends to be accompanied by sadness, forlornness, sorrow, and anxiety. Remarkably, the experience of loneliness can be stopped by choosing to give love and care to others rather than seeking to get love and seeking to be loved. This is a proactive stance and it goes against the idea that the lonely person is a victim of circumstances.

> *It is in giving that we receive and*
> *it is in pardoning that we are pardoned*
> *St. Francis*

In giving, says the prayer of St. Francis, we receive. In loving we are loved. *Alcoholics Anonymous* knows that it is in helping others, one is helped. These are all strategies of overcoming the inner contraction of loneliness and isolation. *All of these strategies work because they help dissolve the background story that you are alone and unloved and the contraction immediately associated with the story.* Releasing ourselves from the story of loneliness and its companion of psychophysical contraction, is the solution to loneliness.

When someone speaks from within the experience of loneliness, more often than not, the voice that is heard is the voice of the frightened, grieving, and abandoned inner child. Loneliness is typically the experience of the inner child who has no one to turn to, carried forward into adult life. In the state of loneliness, the inner child feels unseen, uncared for, unloved, and helpless in some fundamental way to care for itself and its needs.

In understanding that the problem of loneliness is ultimately not coming from the world, I believe that it is helpful to see that when you are caught in loneliness, it is usually you who has tightened up inside and has closed off your own experience of love in yourself and toward others. It is you who has stopped being there both for yourself and others. It is you who does not honor or serve your own needs or the needs of others. It is you who has abandoned your own care and have rejected yourself even though this rejection appears to come from others.

*People are lonely because they*
*build walls instead of bridges.*
*Joseph F. Newton*

If someone has rejected you and you are in the lonely mindset, you often go into agreement with that rejection and wind up regarding yourself in the same unlovable light as you think other regards you. When you are lonely, you often are unaware of how you have isolated yourself, have withdrawn your love, and stopped reaching out to others. This self isolation is typically done to protect yourself from being hurt.

*If you are lonely when you are alone,*
*you are in bad company.*
*Jean-Paul Sartre*

Believing the thoughts that create loneliness is what creates and perpetuates the experience of loneliness. The irony of the lonely person is that as you close yourself off from your own experience of love and hold back your own love for, and interest in others, others do the same in kind toward you.

In the Disney movie *Pollyana*, the young heroine could have suffered from great loneliness and grief. She was an orphan, who had recently lost her beloved father. She was sent to live with an overtly uncaring aunt. Instead of entering in to the typical story of the abandoned and unloved child, she played the *glad game* and perpetually asked herself what she could be grateful for in any situation she was in. While I don't pretend this is the quick answer to loneliness, her triumph in the movie is a moral lesson in the power of changing your thinking and not indulging in the typical thinking of being a victim cast aside and unloved.

*Paradoxical Relaxation* can play a very important role in becoming free of loneliness. *Paradoxical Relaxation* is most helpful in dealing with loneliness when you understand that your loneliness is coming from your own thinking and its related inner psychophysical contraction and not your outer circumstances.

Love is our inner experience when we don't interfere with this experience through thinking that creates fear and self-protection. Getting good at the practice of *Paradoxical Relaxation* may help you to release yourself from loneliness.

# Chapter 3

## *On the shoulders of giants: the background of Paradoxical Relaxation*

## The work of Edmund Jacobson

In developing *Paradoxical Relaxation,* I stand on the shoulders of those with whom I have studied including Jean Klein, Jim Simkin, Yasutani, Erik Peper, Larry Bloomberg, Alexander Lowen, Alan Leveton, and those whose work I have studied like Roberto Assagioli, Fritz Perls, Byron Katie, and others.

*From all of my teachers, I became wise.*
*Psalms 119*

One of the most important influences for me in learning relaxation came from my studying with Edmund Jacobson. Jacobson is considered the father of relaxation therapy in the United States and his method of Progressive Relaxation has been used in one form or another throughout most of the 20th century. Over the years, many research studies have been done on the effect of Progressive Relaxation on conditions ranging from constipation to ringing in the ears. Despite much misunderstanding about Progressive Relaxation, even by professionals who use it, Jacobson's method has stood the test of time.

Jacobson was born in 1888 to a middle class family in Chicago. A brilliant student, he graduated from Northwestern University in two years. At the age of 18, he attended Harvard University. He taught physiology at the University of Chicago and later went to Rush Medical College where he received his MD.

Jacobson related that when he was eight years old, a fire broke out at an apartment house owned by his parents in turn of the century Chicago. Tragically, a close friend of his parents was killed in the blaze and his parents became distraught and hysterical over this shocking loss.

The level of his parents' upset deeply disturbed the young Jacobson. He reported later in his life that at the time of the fire, he vowed never to get upset the way his parents had gotten upset. This desire to remain calm and relaxed stayed with him through adolescence.

Later, when dealing with his insomnia as an undergraduate at Harvard, he began to experiment with his own methods of relaxation. As he developed a technique that allowed him to go to sleep, he chose to write his Ph.D. dissertation on an experiment showing that tense subjects responded acutely to a stressor (two metal bars clanging), while subjects trained in relaxation hardly reacted at all.

Jacobson's life was devoted to applying the principles he developed to the treatment of many psychosomatic disorders. In 1924, he treated women with *globus hystericus*, a condition in which the patient feels that there is something stuck in the throat. Jacobson documented the narrowing of the esophagus in this condition by capturing images of the esophagus with a fluoroscope. He then trained these patients in Progressive Relaxation and fluoroscoped the esophagus after the relaxation training. Not only were the subjective symptoms resolved, but the fluoroscopic images verified a widening of the constricted portions of the esophagus.

Jacobson successfully treated a variety of conditions with relaxation—a treatment that few of his time could understand

For many decades, the conditions Jacobson successfully treated included hypertension, spastic esophagus, spastic colon, headache, functional cardiac disorders like heart palpitation and arrhythmia, as well as the gamut of psychological disorders including anxiety disorders, depression, and mania. He documented the success of his treatment in the many studies he published. What is perhaps more remarkable is that Jacobson proposed the link between stress and illness many decades before it became fashionable. It is also remarkable that he actually treated patients and conducted scientific research on the subject at a time where there was very little interest and awareness of the relationship between body and mind.

In the mid-1940's, Jacobson wanted to develop a machine that would be able to independently verify the efficacy of his method. There were no reliable independent findings that could indicate whether someone was relaxed or whether there was any change in their level of relaxation as the result of Jacobson's intervention.

In conjunction with Bell Telephone Laboratories, he developed the first *electromyograph*, an instrument able to detect electrical activity in muscles with a sensitivity of up to one millionth of a volt. With this machine, formerly undetectable physiologic effects could be easily and scientifically demonstrated. The *electromyograph* could *objectively verify* whether someone was tense or relaxed and the extent to which Progressive Relaxation had an effect.

Although the *electromyograph* formed the basis of the first biofeedback machine, Jacobson did not incorporate the technological wonder he created as a tool in the clinical setting. He took a position that one could not learn to relax while looking at a meter or listening to a tone. He felt that the very act of looking or listening was tension producing and interfered with dropping into the profound states of relaxation for which he was aiming.

*As with anyone who teaches relaxation, Jacobson's method was one of attempting to teach the ineffable.* He understood that language necessarily used verbs that, even if they indicated that someone should relax, implied some kind of effort. Words tend to be crude and verbs like *relax, let go, cease tension, quiet down, stop tensing* all imply some kind of action, some kind of effort— the opposite of what relaxation is. He was clear that relaxation required that one release effort—that one learns to be consciously effortless in order for the muscles to stop tensing and for the nervous system to calm down.

Jacobson's Progressive Relaxation is the practice of conscious effortlessness. His method was home-cooked and his language was peculiar. He told his patients to "discontinue effort."

The most skillful of words can only point to, but cannot precisely capture, the subtlest aspects of what to do in order to relax

When I was learning how to relax, I wish there would have been a book like this available as I struggled to understand his instructions. Jacobson was not forthcoming with an abundance of detail to guide me through the inner territory in search of becoming still inside. The inner world we must spend our time in when we do relaxation is very subtle. Hariwansh Lal Poonja, a meditation teacher, once said to me that the most skillful of words can only point to, but cannot precisely capture the subtlest aspects of our inner world. He said, "What it isn't can be described eloquently… what it is, is a kind of metaphorical room into which no words can enter…." The same is true for relaxation training.

## The *effort error*

One of Jacobson's real contributions was his recognition that effort cannot abort effort. He emphasized this insight in his discussion of the *effort error.* He was a keen observer of minute tensions and would regularly watch patients doing relaxation and observe muscle tension that would be invisible to anyone else.

His instructions and methods were didactic, authoritarian, and typical of the early 20th century, reflecting the concepts of patient and doctor and student and teacher. The concept underlying his instruction was that you followed the teacher's instructions even though his instructions tended to be terse and often obtuse. The student was expected to scrupulously follow the teacher's instructions. Jacobson's tendency to not pay much attention to how his words might be received by patients and students, in my mind, is reflected in the only book that is currently in print which he perplexingly called *You Must Relax.* If I didn't know what kind of giant Jacobson was, a book with this kind of name and its author would have no credibility to me.

Jacobson practiced relaxation daily for most of his adult life until his death. Watching him do relaxation took my breath away in terms of the radiation of effortlessness he exuded. The confidence he exuded, in his writings, his public talks, and my personal communications with him, transmitted a confidence that could only come from someone who was an expert at what he taught.

Progressive Relaxation was the first comprehensive system of relaxation I know of whose developer walked his talk. Indeed, Edmund Jacobson practiced his own method. One important limitation of Jacobson's method, however, was his tendency to disregard the psychological set of experiences with which someone enters into the relaxation training session.

Jacobson wanted to avoid having anyone confuse his method with reassurance or the transference of the patient toward the doctor that Freud focused on in psychoanalysis. He would tell his patients what to do without offering any reassurance or softness in style. I believe his terseness and lack of supportive language was an overreaction to his concern about the dismissal, invalidation, or trivialization of his method by others.

Finally, because Jacobson was very concerned that his method not be regarded as some offshoot of yoga, meditation, or spiritualism, his language tended to be mechanical and appropriate to the scientific and objective language of his peers. This language was sometimes not helpful, instructive, or accessible to those reading his work.

During Jacobson's time, medicine particularly eschewed any religious or spiritual influence, and any hint that a method was spiritual or mystical made the method suspect among the scientific illuminati of the time. Jacobson was careful to shun any *hint* that his method bore any relationship to so-called spiritual practices. In truth, the method of Progressive Relaxation, in essence, is in the finest tradition of the world's effective wisdom practices for bringing peace to body and mind.

## Progressive Relaxation misunderstood

Edmund Jacobson's method is best known for the least important instruction in his repertoire of instructions, namely the instruction to tense and then relax groups of muscles. Many of those who teach Progressive Relaxation misunderstand the method and think that tensing and relaxing muscles is the most prominent feature in the practice of Progressive Relaxation. This couldn't be further from Jacobson's intention. The purpose of Jacobson's instruction to contract and relax was only to raise the consciousness of the practitioner of Progressive Relaxation with regard to the sensation of slight amounts of tension.

The instruction to contract and relax muscle groups was most significant to those who were most out of touch with their bodies. He told patients to contract and then relax the forearm, for instance, so that they knew how slight tension felt, so that they knew on what they were going to focus and what they wanted to relax. Many people whom he treated could not discern tension in their body other than very gross tension. Contract-relax instructions in Progressive Relaxation are aimed at the sensory re-education of the dullest of students of Progressive Relaxation.

Ultimately what Jacobson called 'residual tension' (the amount of tension that remains after one has tried to relax) was the key to relaxing nervous system arousal. In teaching someone Progressive Relaxation, the teacher finds numerous students whose attention has been so routinely exteriorized that they have great difficulty in even identifying the slight guarding, bracing, or tension that never relaxes (this I will describe later as the *default inner posture* that each of us walks around with).

Jacobson's method of focusing attention on one muscle group in the body using peculiar instructions like *discontinue effort, pull out the plug from the wall,* or *go negative* was his best attempt to get his patients to practice consciously letting go of effort. Jacobson knew that the focus of attention on certain parts of the body was more effective in achieving deep relaxation than other parts of the body. Relaxing the forehead, for instance, had a more calming effect on the nervous system than relaxing the arm.

The part of Jacobson's method that is most profound came from his discovery that the movement of the eyes is intimately involved in visual thinking (visualization) and the muscles of the speech apparatus, namely the lips, tongue, throat, jaw and related muscles, are intimately connected to verbal thinking. He discovered that relaxing the eye and speech muscles permitted the practitioner to slow down or stop visualization and verbal thinking. In this slowing down or stopping of thinking, in this 'non-REM relaxation' which is a way I describe *Paradoxical Relaxation*, the nervous system profoundly quieted down and deep relaxation occurred. For some, the relaxation of the eyes and speech muscles is key to their ability to quiet down.

## Jacobson called the esophagus the 'organ of fear'

Jacobson had a keen interest in the relationship between the reaction of the gastrointestinal tract, anxiety, and an aroused nervous system. He spent considerable time treating patients with what is currently called irritable bowel syndrome (IBS), but in his time was called spastic colon. He had an interest in the effects of relaxation and anxiety on the esophagus. When I first met Jacobson at a lecture he gave, I went up to him after his talk. In the course of our discussion, he told me that the esophagus is the 'organ of fear.' Jacobson felt that a relaxed esophagus and colon could not coexist with anxiety and an aroused nervous system.

After I met Jacobson, I had an experience to validate Jacobson's observations on the GI tract and his understanding that the relaxation of the gut was a key issue in relaxation. In a restaurant where I was having a meal with a friend, while eating a piece of chicken, a very unusual event occurred. Suddenly, at the table next to mine a fight broke out between two men. I noticed that a piece of chicken I had been eating simply got caught in my throat. Part of my body's response to the threat of the goings-on at the next table was my esophagus going into a kind of 'freeze' mode where it stopped processing the food I was eating. A few days before this experience, I had a conversation with Jacobson in which he discussed the reaction of the esophagus to the aroused nervous system's reaction to fear or perceived threats.

## Jacobson was the master of his method

Jacobson was the master of his method. A newspaper reporter who interviewed Jacobson toward the end of his life wrote that she acutely felt the level of her own nervousness through the mirror of being around such a profoundly calm man. Story goes that it was his ability to relax deeply and reduce his metabolic requirements for oxygen that allowed him to stay underwater for several minutes.

I would never have learned relaxation had I not viewed it firsthand from Edmund Jacobson, probably the most ardent and passionate practitioner of his method. The evening that is etched in my mind is my meeting with Dr. Jacobson in the upstairs attic of his son's house in California. He looked at me and said, "I'm going to show you how I relax." He proceeded to say, "I'm relaxing my forehead and face now," then he said, "Now, here goes my neck, shoulders, arms, chest, back, stomach, pelvis, and legs." This he did in the course of a minute or two.

What stunned me as I looked at him in relaxation was that as he sat there, he looked like a corpse. Other than the muscles that held him sitting and the muscles of his heart and breath, I saw no sign of muscle activity anywhere. His flesh just seemed to hang off of his bones.

I found myself face to face with somebody who was demonstrating to me what he was asking me to do. The level of quiet I saw in him aroused the deepest feeling in me of wanting to be able to do what I saw him doing and have what I saw him having. The miracle of it to me was that he was really doing it. I found someone who was the real deal. In that moment, I saw that what Jacobson was teaching was possible. He demonstrated it effortlessly before my eyes. This personal experience with Jacobson was a rare gift to me and continues to be in my life. It is so rare in my experience to find the *real McCoy*.

> It is the relaxation teacher's skill and enthusiasm that inspire the student. Teachers who walk the talk are the only effective teachers of what they teach

Like learning the piano or learning carpentry, I believe it is important to have a real teacher who is a true pianist or carpenter. It is the relaxation teacher's skill and enthusiasm that inspires the student. Imagine if you were learning how to play the piano and your teacher didn't actually know how to play but was teaching you from a beginner's book that she herself was studying. Imagine learning how to use a skill saw from someone who was teaching you by reading the manufacturer's instructions because he had rarely used the saw himself. The teacher's understanding of his instructions must come from his own experience and his clarity about relaxation should be obvious to his students.

## Jacobson's enthusiasm and prolific work in relaxation came from his regular experience of profound relaxation

In remembering Jacobson in that profound state of relaxation, it is clear to me that all the research he had done, the books he had written, and his unflagging enthusiasm for his work were fueled by what I believe were his daily experiences of energy and renewal that came from his regular relaxation practice. I understand this now because I see that the energy fueling my own work and writing fundamentally comes from my own experience of doing my own daily relaxation practice when I regularly have experiences of profound relaxation and peace. Without having an example of someone who really knew how to profoundly relax, I don't think I ever really would have believed profound relaxation was possible or committed myself to doing it in the way that I have.

Teachers who are competent in *Paradoxical Relaxation* must have practiced the instructions they are teaching their students innumerable times themselves. Teachers must be able to reliably quiet down their own nervous systems. Competent teachers must be able to easily negotiate the obstacles that are so difficult for their students. It is primarily a teacher's example that provides the motivation for the student to have confidence to persevere in order to move past the difficult obstacles in learning *Paradoxical Relaxation*.

# Chapter 4

## *Relaxing tension by accepting it*

## The practice of accepting tension

*The main insight of Paradoxical Relaxation is that the relaxation of tension that doesn't easily relax involves the acceptance of this tension.* This is a compelling idea though it sounds oxymoronic. "Relaxing tension to accept it" is a large subject and being able to *practice* it as well as intellectually understand it, marks the difference between the novice and the expert in *Paradoxical Relaxation.*

Accepting tension is a subset of a larger issue called accepting what is

Accepting *what is* seems simple. Accepting *what is* when you are doing *Paradoxical Relaxation* means that if you are focusing on your jaw and there's tension in your jaw, you feel that tightness in the jaw. If it does not fully relax, you don't do anything about it. You just accept it as it is. *What is*, at that moment, is your jaw tightness that won't relax. When you accept tension in *Paradoxical Relaxation* you are also asked to accept any resistance to accepting tension.

When you accept tension or discomfort, you are, again, neither adding anything to, nor subtracting anything from, the discomfort. You are *laying alongside* the tension. You are not doing anything to it except being present and feeling it.

The form of poetry known as Haiku demonstrates the pure intention to accept *what is*. Here are some examples:

*The crisp autumn leaves*
*Rustle softly in the wind*
*And then blow away*

*A warm night and gentle breeze*
*the smell of jasmine*
*heavy in the summer air*

In these poems the poet simply reports his experience of what is in front of him. There is no embellishment, no judgment, no interpretation to what is perceived, no 'spin.' The poet reports *what is* directly.

Releasing yourself from the reflex tendency to move toward what is pleasant and away from discomfort is a major event in being able to profoundly relax

## Choosing *not* to be held hostage by the impulse to move toward pleasure and avoid pain

*Paradoxical Relaxation* is a practice of choosing to make our present experience what we want to have, whether normally we would prefer the experience or not. When we move our attention away from what is unpleasant or painful, in this moment *what is* is an unpleasant feeling inside. That unpleasant feeling inside might be a feeling of tension, pain, irritability, agitation, boredom, or contraction of some kind. The practice of *Paradoxical Relaxation* is the practice of accepting all experience, including what is unpleasant.

In the skilled practice of Paradoxical Relaxation, you choose not to be controlled by your desires or aversions

In accepting tension what we are doing is practicing taking control over the natural reflex to avoid pain and go toward pleasure. We're making a choice *not* to be controlled by this natural desire.

Another way of saying it is that we are choosing to not be controlled by our desires and aversions. Reflexively, we naturally go toward what we want and avoid what we don't want. In *Paradoxical Relaxation,* we are practicing releasing ourselves from the control that our desires tend to exert upon us. In the book *Emotional Intelligence*, Daniel Goleman talked about how children who have been trained early on to postpone gratification do the best in life, whereas children who could not postpone immediate gratification in childhood, in a certain sense, do the worst in life in many different ways. In one sense, what we are practicing in *Paradoxical Relaxation* is the postponement of gratification to gain profound relaxation.

## ***Paradoxical Relaxation* is a practice of entering into a universe where everything is *okay***

The term *okay* came into popular usage in the mid-19th century. It can be defined as, assenting or agreeing, giving approval, giving sanction to, being satisfactory, giving an endorsement. In English, when we say *okay,* we are saying yes rather than no, we are giving our consent rather than refusing consent, we are saying fine, good, passable, acceptable, yes, and let's go on. We are saying *yes* to the presence of what we deem to *be okay.*

When I ask you to regard your tension that does not relax as *okay*, I am asking you to accept your tension. You may however be perplexed when I ask you to *be okay* with a feeling inside that says something is *not okay.*

What does it mean to *be okay* with a feeling that says something is bad and shouldn't be allowed? Indeed, this is a trick in undermining the sense of *not okayness.* This trick does not use force, resistance, or confrontation in dealing with the sense of *not okayness.* While it is a trick, bringing an attitude that something is *okay* must be genuinely felt and cannot be manipulated or contrived. You must find a way to genuinely regard something as *okay* for the trick to work. This comes with practice.

When you feel your inner experience is *not okay*, you put yourself in the peculiar situation of regarding the experience in your body as a danger. This is particularly true when there is pain or real discomfort that remains present in the relaxation session. Your body itself becomes viewed as unsafe and you will quite understandably want to distance yourself from it. While you can distance yourself energetically and psychologically from your body, physically you are stuck in it.

In not *being okay* with your inner experience, you key up your nervous system. You tell your nervous system that you are in a situation in which you do not want to be. You regard being in your body as a danger. Not *being okay* with your inner experience for a prolonged period of time is what I believe exacerbates pain and dysfunction in the body.

The practice of choosing to be okay with your inner experience sends a powerful message to your nervous system

When you practice regarding your inner experience, whatever it is, as *okay*, you send a powerful message to your nervous system to stop secreting adrenaline and the arousing biochemicals of fight, flight, and freeze. *Being okay* with your inner experience *is something that must be practiced. Being okay* with your inner experience gets *easier* the more you practice it. This is a practice of self-soothing, a changed attitude that stops the internal wars that often go on against your inner experience.

The practice of *being okay* tells your nervous system there is no danger. There's nothing to tighten up against. There is nothing about which to be aroused. The paradoxical trick in *Paradoxical Relaxation* is that *being okay* with tension and all that has felt *not okay* inside, when practiced repeatedly, erodes the grip of chronic sympathetic nervous system arousal.

## How does it work to *be okay* with anxiety or tension?

One of the essential instructions in *Paradoxical Relaxation* is to *be okay* with the sensation or tension you've chosen to focus on. How do you do that? How does that work?

*Being okay* with tension requires your willingness to tell yourself that something is *okay* and to *want* to believe it. It is a profoundly personal choice to *be okay* with something and no one can force you into it. This is particularly true when your first impulse is to *not be okay* with the sensation you are focusing on or the anxiety you are feeling.

In *Paradoxical Relaxation* an explication of the inner dialogue of a good student is, "I want to trust my teacher that being *okay* with my tension and anxiety is safe and will help me. Therefore, I'm going to rely on this instruction and trust that it's in my interest to assume the belief that being *okay* with my tension and anxiety will help me."

Accepting tension means you choose to feel tension and do nothing about it

When you accept tension, what you do is feel it and make a choice on a moment to moment basis to do nothing about it. Now relaxing tension that you can relax easily is a no-brainer. When you tense your arm and then can relax it easily, there's no effort involved and there's no need to work with that tension because it dissolves by virtue of a very simple and easy instruction you've given to yourself to relax.

It is the tension that does not relax easily, this *residual tension*, that has to be worked with and accepted. In accepting the residual tension and the discomfort of it (because residual tension does not feel great, though it may not feel terrible), we are letting go of the desire in this particular moment to be more relaxed, to feel more at ease or more whole and complete.

Accepting tension is like holding a baby—you do it by holding attention firmly on the sensation of the tension and giving sensation room to wiggle, move, or change. The tension will usually move and shift over and over again. Doing *Paradoxical Relaxation* involves allowing the shifting and squirming of the tension or other sensation as you attend to it and accept it. Remember the tension is your own unconscious holding which you feel as tension. This holding at first does not know what to do with such attention, as it is typically used to your resistance to it. The instruction in *Paradoxical Relaxation* is to *allow* sensation to simply be there, and allow it to move and shift, release and tighten, relax and squirm. Be present with any tension and accept it like you would hold and accept the squirming of your beloved infant.

Accepting tension is like learning to ride a bicycle—
once you understand the concept, the only way
to learn is to get on the bicycle and push off

Ultimately you cannot learn to accept tension from a theoretical discussion of it. Let's imagine you have never ridden a bicycle. We can say, "Put your leg over the bicycle and sit on the seat and push off with one leg while the other leg is on the other pedal and when you start falling to the left, lean to the right, and when you start falling to the right, lean to the left."

For those of us who can ride a bicycle, it is clear that these instructions will not go very far in teaching you how to ride a bicycle. In the end, the only way to learn how to ride a bicycle is to get on one and ride it. Knowing this, parents will often teach their children how to ride a bicycle by letting them get on the bicycle while the parent runs along side of it and holds it upright. Training wheels are sometimes used as a replacement for the parent running alongside the child. While it usually is important to have a coach who is practiced in the skill you wish to master, all such skills are ultimately learned through direct experience. So it is with *Paradoxical Relaxation.*

## Accepting tension includes accepting your limitations to accepting tension in any one moment

In attempting to follow the *Paradoxical Relaxation* instructions, it is helpful to conceptualize that there is this *object* called tension that you want to accept. However, simply understanding the relaxation instructions this way will not get you very far. Accepting tension must include what goes along with it—namely, your resistance, your fear, your difficulty focusing, etc. We want to feel the tension and anxiety, accept them, and accept the way we are best able to accept them, which at the beginning of relaxation training is not so skillful.

For example, if we are only partially able to accept tension, then we want to *be okay* with the limited way we are able to accept this tension.

If we can only receive the sensation in a very limited, contracted way, that needs to *be okay.* This is another way of talking about allowing the resistance to accepting the tension. We are accepting our own tension and equally accepting the limited way we are accepting the tension.

When I say that the whole process of *Paradoxical Relaxation* is accepting tension, I am in the larger sense saying that it is about accepting how I am able or not so able, in any particular moment, to carry out that acceptance. *If there is a limitation in my carrying it out, I want to be okay with that and allow and accept my limitation too.* I want to practice not being frustrated, irritated, or disappointed in how I am carrying out the relaxation instructions in any one moment.

> Becoming more skilled at Paradoxical Relaxation means noticing over and over again the 'no' inside you and accepting it

The way I see it, all tension that doesn't relax is a statement of 'no.' Relaxation is a statement of 'yes.' The *no* in you refers to all of the obstacles in you that don't cooperate with the instruction of accepting tension or anxiety.

All resistance, aversion, attachment to an outcome that arise as you do the relaxation must themselves not be resisted if you are not able to let them go. Distractions that take you away from your focus in the relaxation session—all of what pulls you or interferes with your focus—must be permitted to exist without pushing them away, going toward them, or being upset that they are present in the first place. In this way, acceptance means leaving the resistances inside you alone and ignoring what draws your attention while doing the relaxation.

Paradoxical Relaxation is resting with doing nothing - it is the cultivation of not doing

*Paradoxical Relaxation* can be seen as a practice of resting with doing nothing. In this society that so highly values getting things done, *Paradoxical Relaxation* is an anomaly because it is the cultivation of the ability to *rest* with *doing nothing.* It is the cultivation of hanging out and being comfortable not doing or accomplishing anything. Often anxious patients that I have seen who tend to be addicted to always doing something, struggle with the idea that relaxation occurs by cultivating the ability to rest with doing nothing. Paradoxically, the ability to profoundly relax is prized as one of the highest achievements of the practitioner of relaxation even though there is nothing palpable or material to show for it. The ability to relax is something that no one can take away from you and it is an ability that no one can give you. Yet, if a longer, happier, and more peaceful life is the consequence of *Paradoxical Relaxation*, such an ability carries a value that no material accomplishments can rival.

The ability to relax is something that no one can take away from you and it is an ability that no one can give you

When you are resting, you are ceasing from doing. In a certain sense the phrase 'rest with tension' is an oxymoron, a contradiction in terms, because 'rest' means becoming quiet, being in repose, ceasing action, and moving from doing to being. As tension is obviously a static state of contraction, the words, 'rest' and 'tension' are usually not used together. The instruction 'rest with tension' then is used for this very reason. To rest with tension, you not only have to focus on the tension and feel it, but focus on it and feel it in a state of rest.

## Justness: understanding what it means to *just* feel the sensation

We use the term *just* frequently, but rarely think about what it really means. The terms *just, merely, barely, only, simply* mean nothing else, just that. To accept tension means to feel only the tension and nothing else connected with it—nothing less than, nothing more than.

Justness means this and only this, this and nothing else

Letting go of the outcome means that in the moment, you are *just* feeling the sensation of the tension and not focusing on whether you like the tension, whether you don't like it, whether it's getting you where you want to be or not. It bears saying that the practice of accepting tension means resting your attention on and experiencing *only* the sensation of tension and nothing else.

Resting attention only on the sensation of tension does not mean that other sensations, thoughts, and feelings will not be present in the periphery of your attention. Indeed, thoughts, feelings and sensations that you are not choosing to focus on will often continuously pass in and out of your awareness. The task in *Paradoxical Relaxation* is to stay focused on the sensation you've chosen while allowing these peripheral stimuli to pass in and out of your awareness.

Doing this is not unlike sitting in a booth with a friend at a busy restaurant. As people come and go and with the movement and bustle around you, there is a temptation to take your attention away from your friend to look at what's going on around you. Being a polite and considerate friend, you will tend to resist this tendency to look all around and instead stay focused on the conversation with your friend even though you are aware of the distractions on the periphery of your attention. In *Paradoxical Relaxation*, the restaurant is your mind, the distractions are the thoughts, feelings, and emotions going on in your mind, and your friend is the sensation you have chosen to focus on.

## Faith and patience

Practicing *Paradoxical Relaxation* is practicing being content with what you have in the moment. The trio Crosby, Stills, and Nash sang a famous lyric, "If you can't be with the one you love, love the one you're with." In *Paradoxical Relaxation* "the one you love" is ease and comfort. "The one you're with" is often tension and discomfort. Being present with "the one you're with" and letting go of grasping for "the one you love" cannot be done without patience. Patience requires the postponement of gratification.

Acceptance of tension gets easier as you practice it

What does it mean to accept tension? In short it means the following:

1. To bring your attention to the sensation and feel it
2. To choose to do nothing about it
3. To coach yourself into staying focused on the sensation without fighting it or running away from it
4. To choose an attitude which says that it's okay for the tension to be there or not be there

What defeats most people in learning relaxation is that they don't know what to do with what doesn't feel good inside

*What defeats many people who want to learn relaxation but ultimately give up on it is that they don't know what to do with what does not feel good inside during the relaxation session.* They are immediately looking to feel better. So, they close their eyes, they go inside and there's an inner wiggling and struggle to get out of the feeling.

I have learned that in order to move out of what does not feel good in a relaxation session, I have to start with being present with the feeling. If I try and just leapfrog over what does not feel good inside me, my relaxation remains stalemated and I lose. The relaxation does not occur. Understanding this took me many years.

If you were to close your eyes now and bring your attention inside, your inner experience at this moment may not be exactly what you want. You may want to feel light, loose, joyful, animated, happy, quiet, blissful, or peaceful inside, but you may find that when you close your eyes and go inside that's not exactly what your experience is. When you do *Paradoxical Relaxation*, in the moment that you begin it, when you close your eyes, lie down and bring your attention inside, the real work is to bring your attention to a particular sensation, usually the sensation of tightness, to relax it as much as you easily can, and then when it does not relax anymore, your job is simply to feel it being tight.

As you feel that particular sensation in your jaw, for instance, you might notice on the periphery of your attention that there are sensations that might not feel so good in your head, neck, arms, chest, stomach, pelvis, or legs. You may feel emotionally stressed or sad or angry or fearful. Those sensations and emotions are going on in the moment and the best way to not have them impede your relaxation (and make them disappear) is by acknowledging and accepting their presence.

The fastest way to escape from the discomfort of muscle tension inside is to be present with it

I found in my own practice of *Paradoxical Relaxation* that in order to help myself feel better I had to be willing to feel any uncomfortable sensation inside me and recognize my unconscious inner wiggling and struggle to get away from it. This recognition of inwardly trying to get away from what didn't feel good inside, and allowing that too, helped the discomfort dissolve. What I have come to see is that the paradoxical truth about freeing myself from the unpleasant means I must recognize the resistance in me toward the unpleasant and allow it. I must allow both the discomfort and the inward fidgeting or 'arguing against' or 'pulling away from.'

The key is to notice and observe the tendency inside yourself to want to withdraw and move away from what does not feel good. This noticing is usually instantaneous. Once you can neutrally observe this tendency, then you must simply rest your attention in the presence of sensations that do not feel good. The student of *Paradoxical Relaxation* must be willing to have an attitude of, "If there is nothing I can do about this unpleasant sensation, then I am simply going to focus on how it feels." *Again, this is what it means to accept tension: feeling tension without having to do anything about the tension.* In accepting the tension and the discomfort surrounding it, it is most likely to relax.

## Practicing non-resistance

Accepting tension means practicing non-resistance to tension. We practice resisting nothing and permitting everything. It is when we practice not resisting our resistance that it is most likely for our resistance to soften or disappear. We practice not trying to stop anything, but instead allowing everything in our experience in the moment.

You give it up to get it

Giving up the outcome means you are just feeling the sensation of the tension and not acting out whether you like the tension, whether you don't, whether it's getting you where you want to go or not. Something other than the experience of the tension, like your desire not to feel it or your judgment that it is bad, adds to the sensation of tension you want to not feel. The practice of accepting tension means focusing on and experiencing *just* the tension and nothing else. When you can't let go of your sense of aversion to doing this, you do your best to allow this too.

## *Being okay* if nothing happens during a particular relaxation session

The best attitude to have when you lie down and do a session of *Paradoxical Relaxation* is that you sincerely choose to *be okay* if you don't relax at all during the session. When I suspend my desire to relax during any particular session and am willing to accept whatever is going on in the moment, on a moment by moment basis during the session, whether my nervous system quiets down or not, I am more likely to relax.

It is best to come into the relaxation session with a strong intention to follow the instructions while expecting nothing

There have been many moments in which I felt very tense and up tight and my (usually unspoken) sense was that there was no way anything could happen that would allow me to relax. It took me a long time to notice this sense of 'nothing is going to happen here to allow me to calm down' and to proceed earnestly and energetically in following the relaxation instructions anyway. I would have the sense I was hired to do some kind of thankless job, that I was going to get nothing out of it, and I was going to do this job (which meant continuously resting attention in sensation) with the idea that there would be no reward in it. I was just going to do it full speed ahead with all my intention and energy. I found that by committing myself to what in the moment appeared to be this thankless job of following the relaxation instructions, without my even noticing when it happened, I would regularly enter into the most quiet and delicious relaxation. This is the rule of my experience now.

Therefore, I propose to you that it is best to come into the relaxation session with no expectations. Part of the attitude that I found to be essential in my ongoing practice of *Paradoxical Relaxation* is sincerely and earnestly coming into the relaxation session *from the very beginning* with no expectation of anything. No expectation of feeling better, of relaxing, of anxiety or symptoms going away, of anything at all. When I am willing to embrace this attitude where hankering for gain is renounced, deep and profound relaxation is most likely.

In order to deeply relax using Paradoxical Relaxation, you have to let go of your attachment to being relaxed

## Verbs that best communicate how you focus your attention on tension in order to accept it are few and far between

Over the years I have explored different words and which words best communicate the concept of accepting tension without implying an action or doing. In the past I have used words like 'feel the tension,' 'relax around it,' 'cozy-up to the tension.' I have considered the words 'embrace' or 'welcome.' These words, however, tend to imply being proactive in some way in terms of what is being accepted.

I have come to use several words that have been the result of years of exploring the best language to use in the instructions of *Paradoxical Relaxation.* It may not feel like the words are particularly notable but, in fact, it has taken me a long time to find and use these words and I like them the best. Ultimately, 'accept tension,' in my mind is not the best way to instruct someone in accepting tension. It's not the best phrase to use because, again, 'accept tension' means doing something in relationship to the tension.

I have found that the best phrases to use are 'rest with tension' or 'feel the tension.' The word 'rest' is the least action-implying of verbs. In my mind it is better than 'welcome', 'embrace,' or even 'accept' or 'relax' which are all verbs that imply doing something. In fact, when you rest with tension or you feel tension, I believe you are most likely doing what I am intending you to do when I say 'accept tension.'

In the Middle Ages, when a castle was attacked, the best way to make the castle vulnerable was to dig under the corners of it to remove the support. This was referred to as 'undermining' the castle or digging a mine under the corner walls. The effect of truly resting with tension is the undermining of it. When you bring non-resistance and permission for the tension to be present, in my experience, it is most likely to melt away. The exquisite trick here, though, is to rest with it and have no intention whatsoever of undermining it.

> Resting with tension does not mean resting the tension itself—it means feeling the tension and resting with it

Resting with tension means you do your best to feel the sensation of the tension while you rest as you feel it. You consciously bring repose and rest to what is not restful, to what is tight and tense and contracted, to a part of you that you can't seem to let go of. You bring a state of conscious rest to what is not restful, to what is not at ease.

When you rest with tension, you honor it. You allow it to be present and have an existence of its own without criticizing it, judging it, or wanting to get rid of it. When you rest with tension, it means that you allow it to be the way it is and let it relax on its own terms in its own time. Sometimes I will suggest that people rest with the sensation of tension and leave it alone. Let it have its own separate existence. Resting with tension means that you have faith that it's okay to not intervene in what is troubled, contracted, disturbed, tight, and closed in you.

If you imagine a cat that fell asleep curling up next to your leg, the cat is in a state of rest while it is feeling your leg. The cat is comfortable. In its repose, the cat is not asking you or your leg to do anything or be any other way. It is resting while feeling your leg. It is happy doing this.

Resting with tension is the same principle. You feel the tension and curl up next to it, getting as comfortable as you can with it. You don't demand it be different. You simply rest while feeling it.

## Resting *with* tension is distinct from *trying* to relax tension

Resting with tension is leaving the tension alone and permitting it to have its own existence. Resting with tension means allowing the tension to shift and either get more tense or to relax or to remain the same. It's very important when you are doing *Paradoxical Relaxation* to release an attachment to having the tension relax. *You have to sincerely give up the trying to relax* and rest with the experience of tension.

## The dead-end of *trying* to relax

It is a dead-end to *try* to relax. The novice who *tries* to relax usually remains stalemated in the effort and won't even understand why they are stalemated. I remained stalemated for many years as I subtly *tried* to relax. I did everything I could to kind of 'sneak my way around' the tension that was there. I finally got it. A thunderbolt finally came to me one day and I got the idea, "What if I give up *trying* to relax? What if I give up trying to feel better and instead just feel what I'm feeling and just feel this tension that I'm feeling as it is, with no intention to get it to be different?" This is what Jacobson had said so clearly in his discussion of the effort error, but I hadn't understood how to apply this concept when I was deep in a relaxation session. Then it happened. Boom! The area that I continued to feel, but stopped trying to relax, relaxed. It was remarkable. This is typically the experience when you get good at resting with tension and thereby accepting it. When you rest with tension and completely, totally and absolutely give up trying to get anywhere in that particular moment, relaxation most likely occurs.

In some people, resistance to accepting tension exists because it triggers the idea that accepting tension may mean that it will never go away

At some level, some people resist accepting tension because they are nervous about letting go of control over the tension. But the paradox here is that when you let go of control and just rest with it, the tension is most likely to release.

It is not uncommon for people who are doing *Paradoxical Relaxation*, particularly if they are doing it because of some physical condition or *anxiety state*, to be afraid that accepting the tension means is that they have given up really doing something about the problem and that it is never going to go away. It is not uncommon when I ask people who have other anxiety-related conditions to accept the tension and rest with it, that they have a sense of dread that accepting it means that their condition or their anxiety is going to stick around forever. It's important to identify that fear. If there is any concern, even in the dark recesses of your mind, that accepting tension is somehow dangerous because it means that you've given up, then it is very important to identify those thoughts. In reality it simply is not true that accepting it means it is never going to go away. Actually, when the tension is accepted, it makes it most likely that the tension, and associated symptoms, will go away.

## Getting good at resting with tension

When you first lie down, close your eyes, and turn your attention inward toward the tensed place you have chosen to focus on, your ability to focus your attention on the area will tend to be shaky. The attitude of resting with the tension once you've located it tends to be awkward and perplexing. The novice typically has to deal with micro-reactions inside—reactions of frustration or anxiety—as he attempts to keep his attention focused and to rest at the same time.

When you first begin to do *Paradoxical Relaxation,* it is often an entirely new activity to allow yourself to not be very good at keeping your attention focused. This awkwardness and struggle with keeping your attention focused, with letting go of the outcome, with the letting go of being reactive when you are not able to do what you set out to do, is all normal in the course of learning this method.

In the larger picture, as you get better at *Paradoxical Relaxation*, strangely you get better at forgiving yourself for not being very good at it. It is this continual forgiveness for not always getting it right and not being very good at implementing the instructions, that makes you more skilled in the method and ultimately in resting with tension.

Resting with tension means getting comfortable with anxiety and discomfort

Resting with tension very often means resting with anxiety. Anxiety is essentially a fear response, a biological reaction to some sense of threat. Resting with tension is transcending the reflex to fight, flight and freeze, substituting it with rest and repose. Resting with anxiety is not part of the reflexive programming of survival and it is for this reason that it must be practiced until it becomes automatic.

Being able to rest with what does not feel good inside of you is a milestone

Learning to allow whatever inner experience you have in the moment you begin relaxation is a major accomplishment in someone's life. To be willing to rest with and to be with that which does not feel good inside you is a turning point in your relaxation practice. *In Paradoxical Relaxation, we practice allowing the experience of what does not feel good as a way of getting to the place of what feels good, of what feels easy and pleasant and loose and pleasurable. The paradox of moving from feeling crummy to feeling good is that you have to start with what feels crummy.*

## At the beginning of instruction in *Paradoxical Relaxation*, it is generally better to focus on an area of tension that is free from pain

I do not suggest that someone who is in pain focus directly on the pain. Certainly for the first several months of *Paradoxical Relaxation*, I think it is best *not* to focus on the area of the body producing the greatest symptoms. For example, when someone suffers from pelvic pain, or headache, or TMD, I don't suggest that they focus on their pelvic pain, head pain, or jaw pain.

The reason I don't suggest this is that it is far more difficult to practice the basic principles of *Paradoxical Relaxation*—the principle of feeling the sensation, resting with it continuously, and doing nothing about it—when there is a deep yearning to change what is being focused on. At first, it is far easier to focus on tension in an area that is not problematic like the jaw if one has pelvic pain, the forearms if one has headache, or the shoulders if one has jaw pain. These are more neutral areas and I have found that it is more instructive to practice feeling the sensation and tension in these areas. Later, when one is practiced in feeling sensation and allowing it, direct focus on the area of pain or discomfort central to one's condition is more workable.

When you practice *Paradoxical Relaxation* for a condition in which you are experiencing physical pain or discomfort, it is important to not focus directly on the pain but allow it to exist in the periphery of your attention. Allowing the pain to exist must include whatever contraction you cannot help, that guards against it. This is an important instruction.

For instance, if you suffer from headache and you have chosen to focus on tension in your shoulders, the pain in your head will come in and out of your awareness even though you are not focusing on it directly. It is important to allow this pain to be present in the periphery to the extent to which you can do this without tightening up against it. Once you have allowed it and you notice there is still a tightening up against it, it is important to allow this guarding or tightening up against it as well.

## Distinguishing foreground and background in *Paradoxical Relaxation*

When you sit or lie down to do *Paradoxical Relaxation*, what is foreground is usually the sensation in and around a tight or tensed part of your body. During relaxation, the intention is to keep the sensation of the tension in the foreground, although when you get distracted, the foreground can shift until you bring your attention back to the chosen foreground. In the background of your attention will be any number of things like your mood, some pain or bodily discomfort, your level of hunger, external sounds, the feeling of needing to go to the bathroom, a nagging worry, and typically a kaleidoscope of thoughts that come and go.

Here is the point. If you are doing *Paradoxical Relaxation* and in the background of your attention you are feeling discomfort, restlessness or pain, and you subtly or even unconsciously resist completely permitting and allowing these background thoughts, states or moods, the subtle resistance may unwittingly stalemate your relaxation. I discuss this in the subject of accepting what is unpleasant.

It is best to acknowledge to yourself the background mood or state you are in and allow it to be okay just the way it is. During relaxation, there is nothing you have to do about your mood or state other than to honor its presence and leave it alone.

## Resting with tension needs to include being conscious of, and resting with, your general mood

What exists in the background of our awareness is our general mood. Anxiety, restlessness, agitation, and frustration are among the kinds of moods that are unpleasant. Relaxation, joy, and cheerfulness are obviously happier and more agreeable moods.

It took me a long time to notice that when I was in a disagreeable mood while I was doing relaxation, I was unconsciously struggling to change the mood through my focus on resting with tension in a certain part of my body. I realized that in resisting these moods, I stalemated my relaxation. When I noticed the subtle struggle I was engaged in, in trying to stop my background discomfort, and simply acknowledged it and allowed it to be present, I relaxed far more easily and quickly.

I learned that I had to be aware of the larger mood that I was in, and be accepting of it in the same way I was accepting of the specific muscle tension I was focusing on.

Being aware and accepting of the part of you that does not want to cooperate with the relaxation instructions is essential

Beginners who are asked to accept tension typically have not owned this instruction. They follow it because they're told to. They are not unlike children who are told to eat their vegetables and they will get dessert… they go through the motions of it, but they are not really behind it. They would far prefer to eat dessert.

When you hear the instruction to feel the tension and accept the mood that you are in, especially when the tension or mood is not pleasant or you are having pain, the efficacy of this practice relies on doing it wholeheartedly, sincerely, honestly, and without reservation. *You have to mean it and be sincere about wanting to be okay with it and allowing yourself to feel what's going on inside as it is in the moment. Unless you do, the trick of accepting tension and anxiety doesn't work.*

Instead of subtly resisting or not being fully behind opening up to the tension and anxiety, what I'm saying is that for it to really work, you have to come into harmony with, and tune into, the sensation of tension, and anxiety and truly have the intention to let it into your pores. You have to inhabit your experience as it is in the moment.

Following the instructions of Paradoxical Relaxation cannot be effectively done with a sullen, disgruntled attitude like that of a teenager being asked to take out the garbage

In a certain way, using another simile, the idea of accepting tension and anxiety is similar to having visitors in your house that you don't particularly want to have. You have to decide that you are going to do the very best that you can do to make these visitors feel welcome. You can't just go through the motions of being polite and inviting the visitors in, because they will experience your distance and reluctance to have them around. They will not feel welcomed or at home.

Your own tension and anxiety need to feel welcome and at home in you. What do you do if you are a visitor and feel welcomed and at home? You relax. The tissues of your body involved in tension, anxiety, and physical discomfort do the same.

There are certain visitors in doing *Paradoxical Relaxation*, visitors like tension, anxiety, feeling out of sorts, pelvic pain, and other kinds of discomforts and pains that, if you had your druthers, you would not invite in. You would say, "Stay out. I don't want you in." But when you see the effect of truly inviting them in and making them feel welcome and at home is that they disappear, it is much easier to put your intention and energy into this paradoxical practice.

# Chapter 5

## *Using Paradoxical Relaxation in Difficult Circumstances*

## *Just like this*

It is one thing to read about the principles of *Paradoxical Relaxation* presented in this book. It's another thing to see these principles in action when someone who has practiced these principles for years is in a difficult situation.

The narrative below comes from a long conversation with Walter, a friend and consultant to my book, just prior to his undergoing brain surgery. I recorded the conversation with the understanding and Walter's ready agreement that I would include it in this book. I have edited this interview to clarify parts of the conversation to make them more understandable and put them in context while carefully maintaining the essence of Walter's thoughts, ideas and inner practice. Walter is an 87 year old man who was diagnosed with a brain tumor. He had been in the hospital undergoing numerous tests as well as brain surgery. As with anyone in his position, he has had to deal with the very difficult issue of how to manage, both medically and psychologically, this potentially fatal health problem.

The reason I asked Walter to share his perspective was because I was so moved by the way in which he was handling this most difficult of situations. As he shared how he was dealing with this situation, I was struck by how what he was saying, so closely coincided with the principles I discuss in this book. In presenting Walter's thoughts, my purpose is to illustrate how the principles of *Paradoxical Relaxation* actually look while applied to a very difficult situation like that of my someone diagnosed with a life threatening illness.

> *It is not easy to deal with being told that you have a brain tumor. My first instinct was fear because I was in this situation that I had never been in before. When I was in the hospital a few weeks ago I had all of these tubes attached to me...things going on and doctors and tests and I really didn't know what was happening. It was scary. What was scary was the unknown especially when it looked bad and ugly. It was not anything I would want. So at first I wanted to run from*

*it—I was not open to facing my situation. I didn't want what was happening.*

*When I got over the initial shock and noticed how much I was suffering inside and how agitated I was, I realized I was inwardly running away from what was going on. I knew running away was unworkable. And instinctively I came back to what I had been doing in my meditation practice for many years—I opened to what was going on.*

*I have known for a long time how important it is to open to whatever happens. If you don't open up to what is going on right now, like having a brain tumor, you won't know how to calm down your fear. You have to face fear in order to calm it down.*

*When I first found out about my brain tumor I wasn't doing that. This brain tumor was like having a demon inside of me. So I began doing what I've practiced for many years— I chose to accept the demon and say, "Come let's be friends." When I did this, as I have often experienced, my fear disappeared. I was no longer separating myself from the demon. I included the demon in my life.*

*The point is that I want to accept what scares me. Because what scares me is only my mind conjuring up all kinds of fears that just tighten me inside and out. When I get lost in my mind, I can't see that my fear is just thoughts and I can't relax into the situation. When I don't accept what scares me I am constantly agitated because I am at war with what is going on.*

*Getting lost in our mind is what ruins us. Over the years what I found is that the best idea for me is to say, to whatever difficulty is happening to me, "Just like this—this is the way I want it. Just the way it is." In my current situation the real question for me has been, "How can I have a brain tumor and stay peaceful inside?" Being peaceful no matter what is going on is liberation. So I just accept it. Just like this. It means really opening up my own heart to myself. I say, "I love you," to myself, meaning I love myself and feel compassion for myself. I want to do what I can to help myself accept the situation rather than fight the situation. I've known for many years it's the fighting that creates my problems.*

*What I want to do is bring the fear into my body, embrace it and say it is okay. It is okay just like this.*

*As long as I accept and don't fight having a brain tumor, I am peaceful. I feel centered. I don't have to fight anything. I'm not doing battle with any demon. I accept what is going on, breath and fill up my lungs with the feeling of love and acceptance and compassion for myself that I have in my heart and then I let out my breath slowly.*

*If I entertain just one thought that what is going on should be any different, it plunges me immediately into anxiety. You can call it hell. The separation between heaven and hell is a very fine line. If I spend time lost in fear or scary thoughts about the future, that's hell for me. And if I find that there is fear about the tumor being here right now and I try to push that fear away, I'm in trouble. I just let the feeling of fear be there and I embrace it—this trouble, this tumor, and everything about it is part of my life right now. Another way to say it is that the little kid in me is scared and conjures up all kinds of fears. So I have been saying to this scared little kid inside of me, "It's all right. We'll manage with the demon when it comes. And welcome it in, invite it to sit down and eat and be friends."*

*If I say, "I only want things this way," if I say, "I only want to be alive right now without a brain tumor," I will be agitated. I don't want to be agitated. So, I open my heart to myself and take things just like this. I really am doing it for me and no one else. Opening, welcoming, embracing, loving—it's the opening to the love and compassion in my heart, no matter what else is going on in me, that allows me to be peaceful. With this open heart I face the brain tumor. Without being connected to the feeling in the heart, you've got nothing. I want to keep my heart open no matter what is going on. And what other people think doesn't matter...all I have to do is be open, open to my own love in my own heart.*

*I want you to know how grateful I am for having this understanding and being able to do this, to be able to accept what is going on the way it is going on right now. It's the great paradox. Embrace fear and it goes away. But most people don't have any concept or idea of doing this—they don't want to be uncomfortable and accepting fear in this way at first is uncomfortable and not what they are used to. At the first sign of being uncomfortable, our culture says, "Take an aspirin."*

*With this tumor and the situation I'm in—with having this catheter inside all the time which is very uncomfortable and having to take ½ hour to put on my pants—I have gotten upset. At times I found myself becoming irritated because it is hard to put my leg into a pant leg while being careful not to disturb the catheter. I have gotten angry at my pants. I have gotten upset with myself because it has been taking me so long to dress because I am used to getting dressed right away and getting on with my day.*

*When I realized I was in a state of agitation about how long it was taking me to get dressed, I immediately decided I wasn't going to allow myself to remain agitated. So, from that moment I decided I was going to take whatever time it took me to dress slowly without getting irritated. If it was going to take all day, so be it. I was not going to allow myself to get crazy about having to take a long time to get dressed. What I ask myself when I am agitated is, "How am I responsible for my agitation?" Agitation is all made up—it is about being attached to things being different from the way things are. Now I stay at peace and everything works out...same thing. I do my best to make it be okay. So it takes me an hour to shower and get dressed...that's just the way it is right now and it is okay with me. Patience with your self is a true act of love.*

*I do my best and take what I get. It's very important to take what you get and do the best you can with it. If I can change what I get, sure, I do. But if I can't, I just take it as it is. That's grace. That's the miracle. The miracle is to be able to accept what is going on in my life just this way....just the way the universe gives it to me at this moment. And the next moment it may be different. If I am counting on the future being better or worse in any particular moment, I suffer.*

*When I was in the hospital, there was a lot of noise, a lot of waking me up, taking tests. I had no privacy and people came in whenever they liked to poke and prod me. It was no fun. I could have gotten very annoyed about it all. But I didn't want to be annoyed. I wanted to be in peace. So I said to myself, "Well, look. This is the way it is right now. If they need blood, let them take blood; if they need this, give them this. Just give." I offered no resistance and everything was okay again.*

*When I said to the nurse, "You're such a sweetheart, you must have a lot of people who really care about you," she said, "You'd be surprised. There are people who curse me." And though it was hard to believe, I could understand it. The people who curse her are in a situation like I was in where they're being awakened, they're annoyed, they're angry and they take it out on the nurse. That's what creates the problem. They're agitated and worried and angry all the time. So they blame others. They are fighting their situation. They are not accepting it. That is a formula for suffering.*

*When I noticed my own agitation and I noticed I had become upset when people woke me up for something, I immediately said to myself, "Just like this." Wake me up as much as you like. I relaxed and became giving so that the nurses didn't have to struggle with me. I didn't want them to struggle with me.*

*Managing my agitation is strictly internal. I look to me to calm myself. Really, what else is there to do? Go to a therapist to tell them my story and they're going to fix me? No. I turn inside.*

*My job is to take care of myself. I have been practicing taking care of myself for a long time. It is everybody's job to take care of themselves because nobody else can. You have to practice taking care of yourself and taking care of yourself is all about your viewpoint. It is all about practicing a viewpoint that makes you peaceful. Dealing with this tumor is my practice now. I'm just practicing how to be peaceful and take care of myself in this situation I am in. That's all it is. And it is beautiful.*

*Here is what is amazing. I wouldn't want it to be different. I mean, if I could get it to be different, if I didn't have the catheter, if I could just take a nice walk or swim, it would be wonderful and I would make that happen if I could. But right now I can't make it different. And so I choose to be fine, to be happy with the way it is. It is amazing for me to hear myself say that I am truly happy the way it is. I actually would say I'm joyful. I have this sense of great love for myself. I feel connected to the whole universe and not separate from it. It's all because, for now, I am accepting my life this way.*

*I don't know if you've noticed what I do when I'm a little bit inundated with stuff. I'll just stop for a minute and focus on my breath, take a deep breath and all of a sudden all that tension just disappears. When I accept things this way, not any other way but this way, I relax inside and immediately my whole body relaxes and then there's no agitation and no fear.*

*I know I can't change this situation I am in overnight. It's a process. It came as a process, it will go as a process. So, this brain tumor is what I got. What am I going to do? If I fight it, I aggravate myself. If I become worried about it, I suffer. I've learned that if I want to be peaceful I must take my life the way it is, just like this.*

*Most important, I don't want to live in fear. If I live my life right now the way it is—just like this—if I accept the tumor, I calm down. I embrace it and say, "Fine, I want it to be okay this way." I can't do anything about the tumor right now. So I need to be patient, loving, and appreciative of my own suffering. I want to appreciate and feel compassion for my own suffering. I don't want to run from it.*

*I have practiced all of this in meditation for many years. It actually feels quite natural to me to be doing this. Look, I have very little control over the future. That's just the way it is. I have no plan that something in the future is going to change things. I have no idea if I'm going to get better or not better. All I know is that this is the way it is for me right now. I don't know what it will be 10 minutes from now but whatever comes, I'll deal with it.*

*When my mind goes into the future, there is agitation immediately. I don't have to wait two seconds. My mind, right away, goes into overload. So I do my best to keep my attention present in the moment. When I don't, I get a signal right away. I get nervous, I get agitated, I get worried. I don't want to go there. So, just like on a computer, I delete the thought about the future.*

*In other words, what I'm doing is opening to the universe and saying to the universe, "You tell me. What have you got? Show me what you've got." The universe says, "I got this, I got that..." I say, "Okay, let's do it." In other words, I want to play the game, whatever the game is, I want to participate in the game. I'm not looking to make a different game or a better game or a worse game. Just like this. If it is raining, I practice wanting rain. If it is sunny, I practice wanting sun. Really, it's a paradox. Once you get the knack of it, it is such a wonderful way to live.*

*The knack is accepting things as they come. Then there's very little agitation. You can be calm. You can trust. I am practicing a certain trust that the universe knows exactly what I need. I don't have the answer. I have no idea what the next moment is going to be. So whatever the universe dishes up, that's what I want.*

*Now it's important to say that if I can change something, that is a different story. I change it. If I can't change it, I go with it. I accept it and I'm peaceful. Going into surgery is no piece of cake but I am just going. I tell myself that I've got all the good guys on my side, so I just close my eyes and have fun. It's the only way to go. Anything less than that is nothing but fear and trouble, agitation and worry. I don't want to go there. Right this moment this is the way it is, so I relax. I have nothing to do, no effort necessary. No effort. Just accept it the way it is and you're free. That's freedom. Liberation comes from not trying to change what you can't change. If there is a hairbreadth's deviation about this, you move from heaven into hell.*

*I can feel my own love and my own heart right now, I can feel it. I feel grateful, true gratitude, for just the way I am right now. Look what's happening just by my being open, resolving my own issue of fear.*

*How do you deal with something like this that comes on suddenly? You've got to have practiced little by little. Even though I have practiced acceptance of the way things are, when this happened, it took me by surprise. I remember the doctor said, "You've got a tumor the size of a peach," and that was the last thing I ever expected. I remember just listening. Then surprise. And I didn't know what it meant.*

*Yes, I do have expectations of some kind in the back of my mind that this is going to eventually blow over because I have good doctors and good support. But I am almost 87, I am not naive and I know there is no guarantee. This could be a permanent situation, or worse. So, my intention is to allow whatever comes in to be alright. At times I struggle with my situation; I'm slow, it takes me a long time to move from here to there, I have this uncomfortable catheter, but this is my life now. I just open to it and this opening releases all the anger, frustration and allows me to just be carried by the universe, like a baby. When I allow what is happening and don't fight it, I somehow feel a great love. I could say it is a great love that the universe has for me, although that may sound strange to hear, that is how I feel. When I allow what is happening and don't fight it I have a sense of feeling connected to every human and everything...I feel no separation.*

*What I tell myself is to be receptive, to be open to whatever comes down. I want to be at peace. The only way I can be at peace is to say thank you, thank you, 100% thank you to the universe for whatever comes into my life. If someone gives you a gift, you can either say thank you or no thank you. I say thank you. Doesn't matter what it is. The universe offers the gift of whatever shows up in my life. And I am playing the game of saying thank you. It is just about opening my heart to what has shown up. This sickness has been a wonderful gift. I am peaceful. I don't have to work or figure out anything... I just receive whatever shows up.*

*When I was in the hospital, a nurse came into my room in the morning and said, "What a beautiful day," while I was lying there after only one hour's sleep. I was not a happy camper.*

*He looked out the window and said to me, "Take a look at that gorgeous city." In that moment I was not in a mood to appreciate the view. I thought that that was easy for him to say. He could appreciate the city because he didn't have a brain tumor. Then I realized, "Man, all I have to do is shift inside to get out of my agitated, disagreeable state." And that is what I did. I didn't want to be in that position of being agitated because I was exhausted. I wanted to see things differently. As I stayed with this thinking, I realized that I didn't want to be stuck in some idea of what I liked and didn't like. What I was dealing with was too big. I wanted to be at peace.*

*Then I remember I took a deep breath and I breathed right into the agitation. And I said, "I want it just like this." And I settled down. It took me a little while but I took a few breaths and I started to get in touch with my own heart and my loving and caring for myself. Little by little, before you know it, I was peaceful. I just felt calm. What arose for me and continues to arise is the experience of the bigness and vastness of the feeling in my heart. And in that feeling, everything is alright. And whenever my attention goes toward thoughts that agitate me, I just don't go there.*

*What I am going to say is going to sound really strange. This sickness has been the greatest gift for me that I could ever imagine. It is very joyful. Amazing. I would never have believed it. What is transformative about this sickness is that it is real. It is right in my face, there is no getting away from it. There's no phoniness, this is not made up. It is something that I can't deny. Imagine if I didn't accept this right now? I'd be a mess. The reality of this sickness has forced me to practice assiduously what I have been practicing for years—there is no room for me to do it half-way. When I do this I experience this great peace.*

> *When you have this attitude of allowing everything, of allowing things to be just like this, you can look at life with a smile and you can sleep like a baby.*

In a certain sense Walter's story is the story of someone who, on a moment-to-moment basis and in a life-threatening situation, practiced the instructions of *Paradoxical Relaxation.* Everything that came into his awareness that took him out of the present moment and into thought, he released himself from. Walter's focus of attention was the feeling in his heart and he rested his attention there and returned his attention to it whenever he was distracted from it.

As I spoke to him in the situation he was in, he repeatedly told me how quiet he felt inside. He was actually quite radiant. He remarked over and over again, in spite of what, to most people, would be a nightmare, that he had been having an experience of peace. In his practice over the years Walter had been able to free himself from his resistance to relaxation. Walter's meditation practice had given him the ability to focus his attention easily. He had often reported to me that even in moments of agitation, when he brought his attention inward to sensation, he would become very quiet very quickly. His ability to control his attention came from his long meditation practice. He was one of the rare individuals I have known who often experienced little resistance to letting go of his thoughts and his fears. This, coupled with his long-time practice of returning his attention back to sensation enabled him to be so remarkable in dealing with his situation.

Walter's story makes calming down even in the most horrendous of circumstances sound easy. His ease came from the many years he practiced the principles described in this book.

Most people who begin *Paradoxical Relaxation* encounter many obstacles to being able to rest their attention in sensation that have been long-resolved by Walter. Most people who begin to practice *Paradoxical Relaxation* must spend extensive periods of time becoming aware of and releasing themselves from their attention caught in fear and thoughts of past and future. As you can see in my Walter's story, he was an old-hand at all of this. In the following chapters, I discuss how to deal with the subtle resistances and impediments to being able to rest attention in sensation and become quiet inside. Indeed, this book and the subject of addressing the resistance to relaxation, is designed to help those new to relaxation training. It can help those with little training in controlling attention to navigate through the subtle and unconscious barriers that typically stymie those who wish to learn how to quiet down inside.

# Chapter 6

## Residual tension and the *default inner posture*

## Relaxing the *default inner posture* is the key to lowering nervous system arousal

The *default inner posture* can be described as an inner pattern of slight, stubborn physical tension associated with an inner attitude of vigilance, fear, and guarding. Surprisingly, relaxing the apparently unremarkable tensions that comprise the *default inner posture* is the key to both lowering anxiety and the arousal of an agitated nervous system. In this chapter, I will discuss the *default inner posture* and the understanding and methodology about becoming conscious of it and relaxing it.

*Human suffering in any way involving anxiety is both a physical and mental event.* The mental and emotional experience that occurs when you are regularly tense or anxious, as in other emotional states, is accompanied by a physical one—a *default inner posture*, a characteristic, conditioned, *slight yet enduring, physical bracing which typically is defensive in nature.* The *default inner posture* usually remains unconscious but can be brought into consciousness by re-connecting with and feeling oneself as the agent of this *default inner posture.*

## Identifying tension in your body

A preliminary exercise in beginning *Paradoxical Relaxation* directs patients to do an inventory of tension throughout the major muscle groups of the body. Forehead, face, jaw, neck, shoulders, arms, upper back and chest, lower back and stomach, pelvis, legs and feet are carefully examined and any tension in these areas is identified. Instruction asks the beginner to find a part of the body (preferably in the upper body) that feels any degree of tension. It does not have to be any great or unbearable tension, just a simple sensation of tension. Tension in the shoulders or neck, however unremarkable, is a suitable area to focus on for the purpose of this exercise, at the beginning of relaxation training. In choosing a tensed part of the body on which to focus, it is important to make sure that the tension chosen is not painful but simply tense.

## It is important to recognize tiny sensations of tension during *Paradoxical Relaxation*

It is important to understand what constitutes tension is the object of focus in *Paradoxical Relaxation* instructions. The slightest, tiniest bit of tension is considered significant even though most people normally would not pay attention to it. Residual tension is the small amount of tension that you can't seem to relax when you first try to relax. It is unobtrusive and unremarkable. You would not pay attention to it unless someone brought your attention to it. You'd certainly never think it was important. *Paradoxical Relaxation* depends on the identification and ability to discern this very small amount of tension.

The relaxation of the tiny, or what is also called 'residual,' tension is the key to reducing nervous system arousal

In Edmund Jacobson's work with relaxation, he noticed that the level of the tension that stood in the way of relaxation appeared to be both very small in one sense, but also a huge obstacle in another. He discovered that when he was able to profoundly relax, what he called achieving "an extreme degree of relaxation," he had released an apparently small degree of tension. When this stubborn bit of tension dissolved away, he was ushered into a state of deep, profound relaxation. He called this small degree of remaining tension *residual tension.*

Relaxing residual tension is the key to profound relaxation

In his book Progressive Relaxation, originally written in 1929, Jacobson described residual tension in the following way:

> *"When the unpracticed person lies on a couch, as quietly as he can, external signs and tests generally reveal that the relaxation is not perfect. There remains what may*

*conveniently be called residual tension. This may also be inwardly observed through the muscle sense. Years of observation on myself suggested in 1910 that insomnia is always accompanied by a sense of residual tension and can always be overcome when one successfully ceases to contract the parts in this slight measure. Residual tension, accordingly, appears to be a fine tonic contraction along with slight movements or reflexes. Often it is reflexively stimulated, as by distress or pain; yet even under these conditions relaxation is to be sought.*

*Doing away with residual tension is, then, the essential feature of the present method. This does not happen in a moment, even in the practiced person. Frequently the tension only gradually disappears; it may take 15 minutes progressively to relax a single part, such as the right arm. The desired relaxation begins only at the moment when the individual might appear to an inexperienced observer to be very well relaxed.*

*When the individual lies "relaxed" in the ordinary sense, the following clinical signs reveal the presence of residual tension: respiration is slightly irregular in time or force; the pulse-rate, although often normal, is in some instances moderately increased as compared with later tests; voluntary or local reflex activities are revealed in such slight marks as wrinkling of the forehead, frowning, movements of the eyeballs, tenseness of muscles about the eyes, frequent or rapid winking, restless shifting of the head, a limb or even a finger. Finally, the mind continues to be active, and once started, worry or oppressive emotion will persist. It is amazing what a faint degree of tension can be responsible for all this.*

*The additional relaxation necessary to overcome residual tension is slight indeed. Yet this slight advance is precisely what is needed. Perhaps this again explains why the present method has hitherto been overlooked. As relaxation advances past the stage of residual tension (chaps. vii, viii, ix, x, xvi), respiration loses the slight irregularities, the pulse-rate may decline to normal, the knee-jerk diminishes or disappears along with the pharyngeal and flexion reflexes and the nervous start, the esophagus (assuming that the three instances studied are characteristic) relaxes in all its parts, while mental and emotional activity dwindle or disappear for brief periods. The individual then lies quietly with flaccid limbs and no trace of stiffness anywhere visible, with no reflex swallowing, while for the first time the eyelids become quite motionless and attain a peculiar toneless appearance. Tremor, if previously present, is diminished or absent and slight shift of the trunk or a limb or even of a finger now cease to take place. Subjects independently agree in reporting that this resulting condition is pleasant and restful if persistent, it becomes the most restful form of natural sleep. No university subject and no patient has ever considered it a suggested or hypnoidal or trance state or anything but a perfectly natural condition. It is only the person who has read a description without witnessing the actual procedure who might question this point."*

## Inner tension that does not easily relax is easily missed

The outside world is familiar to us when we open our eyes and look across the room or across the street. If we are asked where the street corner is, we will easily locate it. Similarly, if we were told to look at our left knee, we would not have any trouble in finding it. If we were to look at our right hand, again, we would not have any difficulty in locating it.

The inner world of sensation, thought, and emotion is not so clear. It is usually subtle and unremarkable. For example, when we close our eyes and direct our attention to the sensation of our neck, while its location may generally be clear, the sensation of our neck usually does not have the discreet boundaries and precise location that appear when we see our neck with our eyes open. In learning *Paradoxical Relaxation*, we practice locating sensations inside the body. Tensing and relaxing a part of the body can be useful in teaching us to locate the tensions in the body while the eyes are closed.

In the beginning of relaxation training, attention is directed inside the body in order to locate tension that does not relax. Patients are asked to feel the tension without trying to modify it or reduce it. The purpose of this initial focus on tension is to help the patient identify slight muscle tension that doesn't relax.

## Cultivating an attitude of receptivity toward slight sensations of tension

There is a quality of attention that can help more clearly locate and relax tension in the body. When patients are first learning *Paradoxical Relaxation,* they are asked to be more receptive than active in perceiving it. They are asked to allow the sensation to come toward them, so to speak, rather than actively reaching out toward it.

To best achieve this receptive attitude, it is important to practice steadying one's attention. Patients are asked to feel the tension in the body without trying to define its borders or its exact location within. Sometimes I use the analogy of a self-focusing camera. The camera is simply pointed in the direction of the object to be photographed. This triggers an automatic focusing of the camera's lens. The photographer simply has to turn this point-and-shoot camera in the direction of the object and everything else occurs automatically.

## Using your attention like a camera

In locating inner tension, attention works like this kind of camera. Point attention at inner tension, sustain it there, give attention a chance to settle down and the sensation of the tension usually comes into focus without effort. I ask patients to tolerate that the sensation they are focusing on may be subtle, vague, and not clearly differentiated. I ask them to take that sensation exactly as it shows up in their awareness.

Again, I ask patients to not be concerned about gaining a sense of the precise boundaries of the tension. The sensations of the tension usually come on their own terms, like the smell of jasmine wafting into awareness on a warm summer night. The scent of jasmine need not be grabbed. As the aroma finds its way into the nostrils, so the sensation of tension finds its way into awareness with the very simple act of focusing and resting attention upon it.

Tightening and then relaxing muscles is simply a sensory exercise in discerning residual tension. In and of itself, it does nothing to facilitate relaxation. The relaxation of residual tension is what Progressive Relaxation was all about. Jacobson said in Progressive Relaxation:

> *"Doing away with residual tension is then, the essential feature of the present method (i.e., the method of Progressive Relaxation)."*

Residual tension is something that is almost unnoticeable. It is the slight tension that we live with and make little or no note of. Often in the clinics we hold, people who are used to ignoring their bodies and being tense their whole lives, dismiss the sensation of residual tension entirely. It is common that they don't even know it is there until they quiet down enough and are properly instructed in identifying it. Until they can discern the residual tension, they tend to flounder in progressing with the relaxation protocol.

Residual tension is typically the expression of an unresolved state of guardedness and self-protection

What Jacobson missed in his brilliant and seminal insight about residual tension was that residual tension is not simply a physical event but the expression of someone's enduring psychological and existential state. I am proposing here that residual tension is a link in the chain of tensions that make up a defensive inner posture that often has endured for many years. It is the underlying residue of someone's unconscious vigilance in the world.

To explain this further, it's important to understand that feelings of anger, fear, sorrow, grief, dread, disappointment, and despair are simultaneously physical patterns of tension and emotional states that are inextricably tied together. Change one, and the other can't remain in place. In *The King and I*, Rodgers & Hammerstein wrote a musical treatise on changing the physical expression of fear to get rid of it. Below are the lyrics to *I Whistle a Happy Tune*:

*Whenever I feel afraid,*
*I hold my head erect,*
*And whistle a happy tune, so no one will suspect,*
*I'm afraid;*

*While shivering in my shoes,*
*I strike a careless pose,*
*And whistle a happy tune,*
*And no one ever knows,*
*I'm afraid;*

*The result of this deception,*
*Is very strange to tell,*
*For when I fool the people,*
*I fear, I fool myself as well;*

*I whistle a happy tune,*
*And every single time,*
*The happiness in the tune,*
*Convinces me that I'm not afraid;*

*Make believe you are brave*
*And the trick will take you far,*
*You may be as brave, as you make believe you are,*
*As you make believe you are.*

In *Paradoxical Relaxation*, the happy tune that is whistled when afraid is the protocol of accepting the tension. In *The King and I,* Anna changes her psycho-physical state of fear by doing her best to change her physical posture (*strike a fearless pose)* and change her behavior *(whistle a happy tune)*. She changes the psychological by changing the physical and behavioral expression of the psychological state of fear. In *Paradoxical Relaxation*, the way we change fear or anxiety is by accepting and resting with it.

## Wilhelm Reich, Frederick Perls and the focus on the body in psychotherapy

The observation that chronic muscle tension is part of an individual's psychological defense system has been part of the model of personality in several schools of psychotherapy including that developed by Wilhelm Reich. Reich worked in Freud's clinic in Vienna in the 1920's, although he later came into conflict with Freudian theory. In his book *Character Analysis,* he proposed that neuromuscular contraction, or *muscular armor,* was an integral part of someone's character structure and system of psychological defense. He described 7 tension rings of muscular armor involved in the suppression of emotion and impulse.

In what became known as Reichian therapy and Reichian-oriented therapy, Reich and his followers used breathing techniques, palpation of chronic areas of contraction and other methods to release the body armor, allow emotional expression, and unblock what he discussed as a kind of energy that has been blocked by such muscular contraction.

There have been offshoots of Reichian therapy including the method popularly known as bioenergetics, written about by Alexander Lowen and others. The focus of these Reichian-oriented methods has been to oil and rehabilitate the body's cathartic machinery that somehow became rusted and non-functional. These therapies aim to release muscular tension associated with psychological defense through techniques that involve release of suppressed emotions. Typically, in a Reichian-oriented session, the patient is instructed to breathe in a certain way in combination with certain interventions of the therapist that support the expression of suppressed emotions. This has often been an effective method in helping patients suffering from a variety of psychological conditions related to emotional suppression. While these catharsis-inducing methods are very different from *Paradoxical Relaxation,* they can be used complementarily when trauma and emotional suppression are issues.

Frederick Perls was a German psychiatrist whose method called *Gestalt Therapy* came into use in cutting edge therapies blossoming in the 1960's and 1970's in the United States. The focus on the physical expression of personality has been part of the Perls' methodology. During a psychotherapeutic session, Perls would often draw the patients' attention to their posture or physical expression and have them embody this expression to tease out the psychological stance that this posture was expressing. His method is known to involve having the patient have a dialogue with different parts of the personality, sometimes expressed in patients physical posture, by having the patient 'put one part of them in a chair' and speak to this part. He would then have the patient switch chairs and respond back. In this way, he facilitated a reconciliation of 'owning' of the disowned parts of the personality. I have borrowed from my experience doing *Gestalt Therapy* in the practice of 're-owning' the residual tension or what I will discuss below as the *default inner posture.* Perls, like Reich, was an innovator, and his psychotherapy, in my view, has made a major contribution to psychology.

In the practice of Paradoxical Relaxation, I am giving the name default inner posture to the pattern of tension that does not relax

*Paradoxical Relaxation* urges no emotional release even though it may come from time to time. It requires no interpretation of intrapsychic events even though insights about one's inner life and motivation can occur frequently. In *Paradoxical Relaxation,* we can work to release ourselves from our *default inner posture* on a daily basis.

We do *Paradoxical Relaxation* to dissolve anxiety by changing our physical posture (*resting attention in sensation*) and changing our attitude (*adopting an attitude of acceptance and compassion)* toward our own experience of anxiety.

As the strategy of *Paradoxical Relaxation* helps the patient release the physical expression of tensions associated with vigilance, guarding, fear, anxiety, anger, and dread, these emotions can arise as the tensions connected to them relax. While this does not always happen, it is not uncommon.

## Relaxing the *default inner posture*

Residual tension refers to the slight amount of tension that remains after you relax as best you can. The *default inner posture* refers to the inner *pattern* of residual tensions—usually a pattern of slight tension associated with underlying self-protective states of vigilance, fear and guarding among others. When you feel the inner posture of your slight holding, as I describe below, the way you hold yourself in the world usually becomes clear. If in fact your *default inner posture* is the physical expression of an ongoing psychophysical state of guarding and attendant autonomic arousal – and if relaxing this *default inner posture releases* you from your underlying self protective state of guarding – it is not surprising why Jacobson observed that relaxing residual tension is the key to lowering autonomic nervous system arousal. Why? Because the underlying self-protective state of guarding arises simultaneously with arousal of the autonomic nervous system. Relaxing this guarding turns down the arousal because they are married to each other.

Making the *default inner posture* conscious means reconnecting with, re-identifying with, or re-owning the slight residual tension that doesn't relax. It means experiencing again that it is *you* who is continually doing the tensing and not something happening to you. When you feel yourself as the one who is the agent of the tension, your *default inner posture* becomes clear. In this section, I want to discuss the *default inner postures* of anxiety, fear, dread, anger, sorrow, grief, despair, guilt and shame.

The *default inner posture* is the physical expression of what is really going on inside of us. It is where we are living. When we strip away all of our distractions and avoidance, the *default inner posture* is how we find ourselves feeling in relationship to life and existence. You can feel this posture as you settle down during sessions of *Paradoxical Relaxation* as attention rests in sensation outside of thinking and distraction. This posture remains in place in the form of slight but chronically held tensions that consistently reassert themselves. The *default inner posture*, when it is protective and fearful, stands in the way of deep relaxation and fully being alive.

The *default inner posture* is obvious as we understand that human beings, in large part, are animals whose bodies are hard-wired to survive. When we are frightened, our bodies tense up to survive. When there is a *default inner posture*, the pattern of tension in the service of survival has been activated and never fully deactivated.

## The *default inner posture* is the physical expression of the core of the personality; dementia, intoxication, and the emergence of the core personality

When someone has dementia, the structure of the brain deteriorates and the normal cognitive processes progressively become impaired. When this occurs, among other changes, there is a process of disinhibition that occurs in which someone progressively becomes less and less able to control impulses. This process of disinhibition means that basic impulses related to others in the world, the impulses of fear, anger, or sexuality come to the fore. This is why the core of the personality, which is our default system of dealing with emotions and sensations, becomes more clearly expressed.

The default mode of the personality can also come to the fore when someone is drunk. In this state, the underlying attitude toward others and the world, the default emotions that someone lives with and the default response to others in the world show themselves more easily without the normal inhibition that occurs when someone is not intoxicated. Thus people are called *happy drunks* or *mean drunks*. Similarly, for instance, you can have someone who has dementia who tends to be happy, cheerful, and loving or someone who tends to be angry, fearful, and paranoid. Like the *happy drunk* or the *mean drunk,* there is the *happy demented person* and the *mean demented* person. Happy and mean are default stances in life that become most clearly visible when there is little ability to disinhibit their expression.

The *default inner posture* is your existential stance toward life under certain circumstances. It is your core stance toward the world expressed in numerous ways, but importantly through an inner set of tensions that remain in place. Under stress, this posture may become exaggerated.

The default inner posture is a psychological and physical state of self-defense that somehow 'got stuck'

*Default inner posture*s can come from childhood and involve painful, difficult circumstances that have not been resolved. So the body remains in a state of readiness, a kind of ongoing default posture of vigilance or defense. For example, the *default inner posture* may exist in response to a fearful reaction to mother or father's abusive anger or an intolerable sense of abandonment that you carry around because you never quite got over certain events or circumstances, imagined or real, to which your body is still reacting.

If you imagine early in life feeling shame or fear or anger or desire that for whatever reason felt overwhelming, the way to stop the overwhelm would be to tighten up physically against it. This defense against feeling what is intolerable or overwhelming is both psychological and physical. I am suggesting here that the way in which these feelings remain suppressed is found physically in residual tension.

Someone's default inner posture is
almost always unconscious

These postures tend to endure throughout life and are almost always unconscious although with a person's willingness and with thoughtful instruction, they can easily be made conscious. Depending on the sensitivity of others or how well they know you, they can see your *default inner posture* even though they might not identify it as such. There are some individuals who appear perpetually glum, worried, angry, or depressed. If you look at the *default inner posture* of these people, you will see certain groups of muscles that are engaged in a certain pattern of holding.

The default inner posture of someone who is
perpetually worried is associated with tension in the
forehead, shoulders, neck, jaw, abdomen, and pelvis

We recognize when someone is out of their *default inner posture* when we notice something is changed or uncharacteristic about their demeanor. Take for instance person whose worry is clear to us at some level even though we often haven't actually named this characteristic. When you examine the pattern of residual tension in this person you will find that, among other muscles, the 'worry muscles' are engaged. It's common knowledge that the forehead furrows when you are worried. The worried *default inner posture* is also associated with tension in the shoulders which are usually raised, tightness in the jaw and neck, tension in the pelvis and elsewhere. Similarly, there are patterns of tension associated with a person who tends to be in an angry inner posture, or a despairing inner posture, or in a grief-stricken inner posture.

When we are close to a chronically worried person, and one day this person seems uncharacteristically cheerful and bright, we might think, something good happened to this person or maybe they are in love. When we examined their *default inner posture* and the pattern of slight (residual) tension that makes it up, the uncharacteristic cheer of our normally worried friend will reveal a certain relaxation of the muscles of their *default inner posture. Paradoxical Relaxation*'s aim is to give individuals the ability to relax their *default inner posture* that is associated with anxiety and other disturbing underlying emotional states.

## The *default inner posture* can relax its hold during intimacy, intoxication, altered states and sleep

The *default inner posture* may relax during intimate contact, intoxication, altered states, sleep. When you are in bed with your beloved, touching and feeling physically and emotionally close, the tensions that guard and protect can drop away. This is certainly why sex sells. Everyone wants to return to the unguarded state in which life is immediate and there is no barrier between you and aliveness. The popular media and the advertising sciences have linked this sense of immediate, open contact with the heart of life with sexual images and allusions and in fact the human psyche responds. Sex does sell because I am proposing it promises the dropping of the *default inner posture.*

Intoxicants also allow guardedness to drop away and can chemically release the grip of the posture of inner vigilance that keeps the joy and immediacy of life at bay. When intoxicants chemically bring about what you can call disinhibition in someone who has not explored their inner life, this disinhibition can include the release of control over aggression and we get to see the side of some personalities that you can call the *mean drunk.*

The programming of the *default inner posture* can also release during deep levels of sleep, only to reassert itself upon awakening. Many people who are guarded and vigilant in their life can relax and let go when they fall asleep, and sleep for many people is a release from the general conditioning of the *default inner posture.* In other words, the unconscious rule is that as long as you are awake you have to stay watchful, oriented and vigilant. Under certain circumstances like sleep, the body's conditioning says it is okay to drop this vigilance.

Paradoxical Relaxation can be described as a practice of resting and re-identifying with the default inner posture in order to dissolve it

**The *default inner posture* can have its origin in unresolved situations of childhood or can simply be the way in which someone has been socialized to life in the world**

Beyond all else, a mother's job is to protect her child from harm. For example, it is a major event in the lives of mothers and children for a mother to let her child walk to school on his or her own without the mother's watchful eye. When that fateful day comes, when the child goes to school alone, all mothers without exception will tell their children to be careful, to watch out for danger so they don't run into the street, or in some way put themselves in the way of harm.

With rare exception, the child hears mother's concern clearly. So here you are, a 5 year old on your way to school by yourself, excited and a little scared at being on your own in a big world. You know that your mother is nervous and somewhere you know that there is danger if you don't follow her instructions about remaining safe. So you are watching out, you are being careful. You are remaining vigilant and guarded on some level. If the muscles in your body were to be examined, there would be some level of tension associated with your intention to stay vigilant, remain safe, and follow your mother's directions.

Your first day of going to school by yourself may be one in which you are actively watching out carefully to remain safe. As the days, weeks, and months pass during which you continue your independent travel out in the world, you continue to comply with mother's instructions, and you soon do so without being conscious of such vigilance. Your vigilance becomes a conditioned way of being in the world. This conditioned vigilance is intimately connected with the physical posture of vigilance which is one form of what I am calling the *default inner posture.*

The formation of the default inner posture
coincides with some children losing their
spontaneity, vivaciousness, and sense of wonder

We have all seen young children who are vivacious, spontaneous and natural lose their spontaneity, playfulness, and ease as they get older. Most of us are delighted to see children who have appeared not to lose these qualities as they get older. The loss of these qualities, again, is both a physical and psychological event.

## Becoming aware of your *default inner posture*

In re-identifying with your *default inner posture*, you are generally moving what has been unconscious to what is conscious. You rediscover not just intellectually, but experientially, that you are the agent of your own contraction. In the immediate experience of reconnecting yourself with this chronic residual tightening, it becomes much easier to relax.

In order to dissolve the *default inner posture,* it is most effective to do relaxation with the clear understanding that the task is to rest *with* the sensation of the *default inner posture* and *not to try to directly relax it.*

In being able to dissolve the *default inner posture,* you are releasing yourself from the imprisonment of your instinctive self-protective or survival response that may have been conditioned early in life. The *default inner posture* needs to be intimately known without judging it. You need to become familiar with it in the way you are familiar with the back of your hand. You job is to become very comfortable in hanging out with it, like an old friend you've known forever.

Becoming aware of your default inner posture is typically a process of re-associating with that from which you have been dissociated

If these slight patterns of tension are fully expressed, a person could not function or be socially appropriate. We usually hide our core posture toward the world although we cannot get rid of it entirely—the contraction remains in the form of the slight tensions that we cannot relax.

Reconnecting with the fact that it is *you* who is doing the residual tightening can be illustrated by having your right hand push against your left hand. If you focus on your right hand doing the pushing, sooner or later you will lose touch with the fact that your left hand is pushing back. Your attention isn't on what your left hand is doing but only on what your right hand is doing. If you then switch and feel your left hand pushing against the right, you reconnect with what you are doing that you lost touch with. Coming back into connection with the residual tension is the same.

## Inhabiting the *default inner posture*

Dissociating from the *default inner posture* is taking attention away from the sensation of the contraction. When you are dissociated, you don't experience yourself as being the agent of your tensions. When you re-associate with it, you 'inhabit' this experience in your body. You enter it. You allow your attention to be present in it. This is like bringing your attention back to your left hand when your attention has been only connected to the sensation of your right hand. You re-enter this holding you have been doing.

Inhabiting what you have split yourself off from requires that you be able to control your attention enough to stay connected. Re-inhabiting your *default inner posture* is like tuning a radio to a certain frequency--you have to tune your attention to the pattern of tension that you rarely tune to tune to tune to. This tuning in means that with steadied attention, you are able to focus on how you are holding yourself in your *default inner posture.* You have to have your attention steadied so that you perceive your posture among all of the competing sensations inside.

## *Default Inner Posture* of Fear

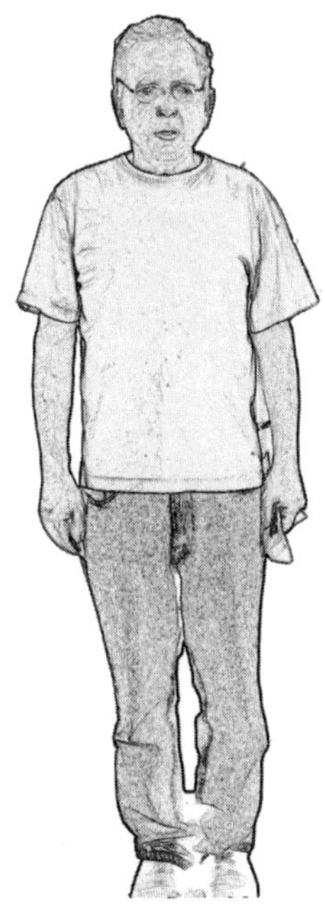

The normal appearance of the *default inner posture* of fear showing unexaggerated pattern of tension in the jaw, forehead, neck, shoulders, arms, hands, stomach, and pelvis

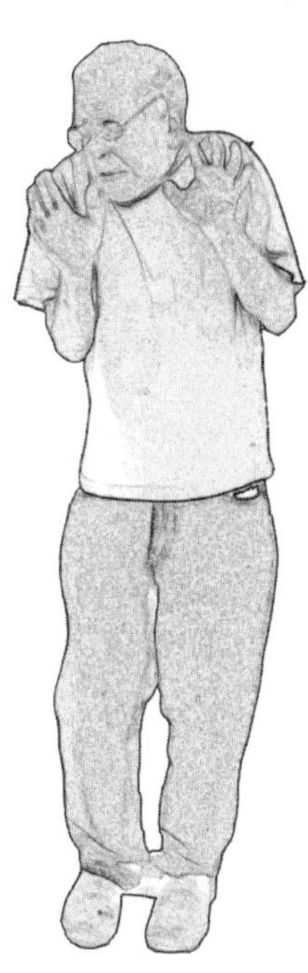

Exaggerated *default inner posture* of fear: clarifying the pattern of muscle tension associated with chronic fear

## *Default Inner Posture of Sorrow & Grief*

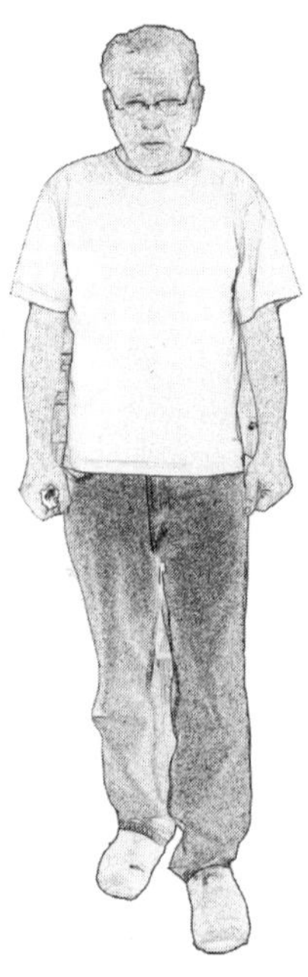

The normal appearance of the *default inner posture* of sorrow & grief showing unexaggerated pattern of tension in the jaw, forehead, eyes, neck, throat, shoulders, arms, hands, chest, and stomach

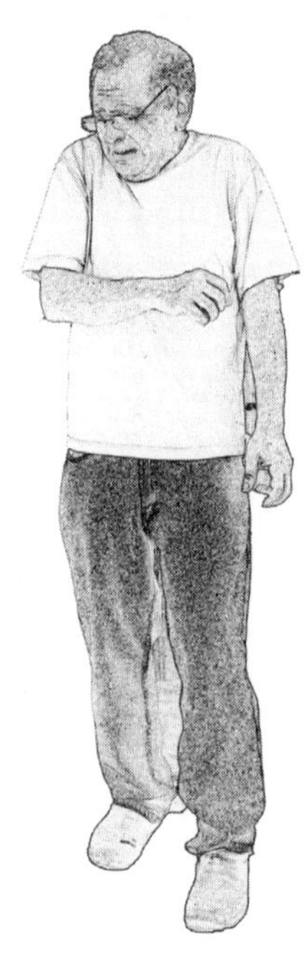

Exaggerated *default inner posture* of sorrow & grief clarifying the pattern of muscle tension associated with chronic sorrow and grief

## ***Default Inner Posture of Despair***

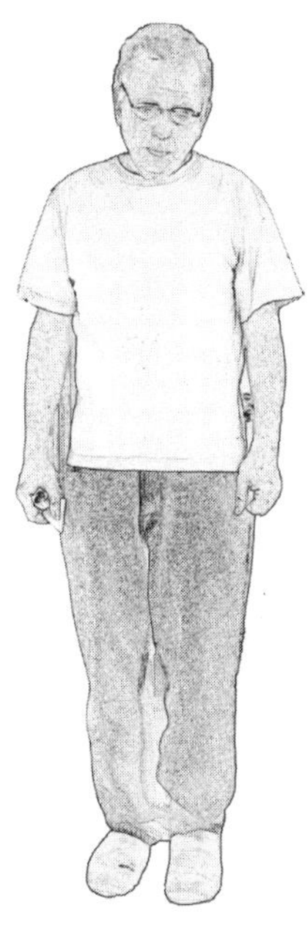

The normal appearance of the *default inner posture* of despair showing unexaggerated pattern of tension in the jaw, forehead, eyes, neck, throat, shoulders, arms, hands, chest, and stomach

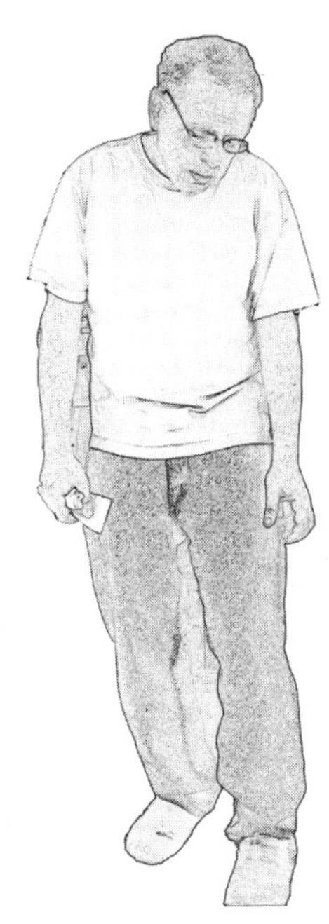

Exaggerated *default inner posture* of despair: clarifying the pattern of muscle tension associated with chronic despair

## *Default Inner Posture of Shame*

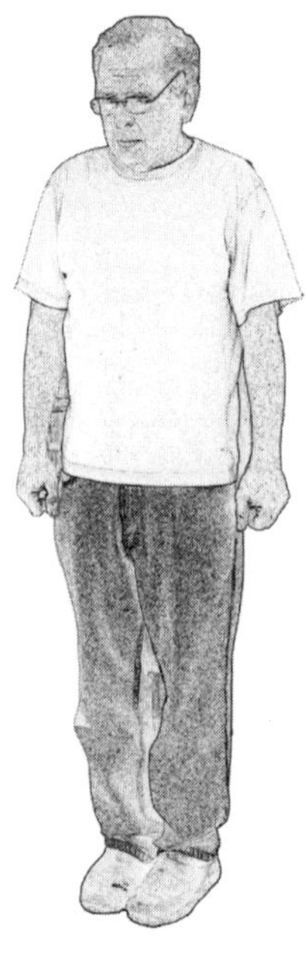

The normal appearance of the *default inner posture* of shame showing unexaggerated pattern of tension in the jaw, forehead, eyes, neck, throat, shoulders, arms, hands, chest, and stomach

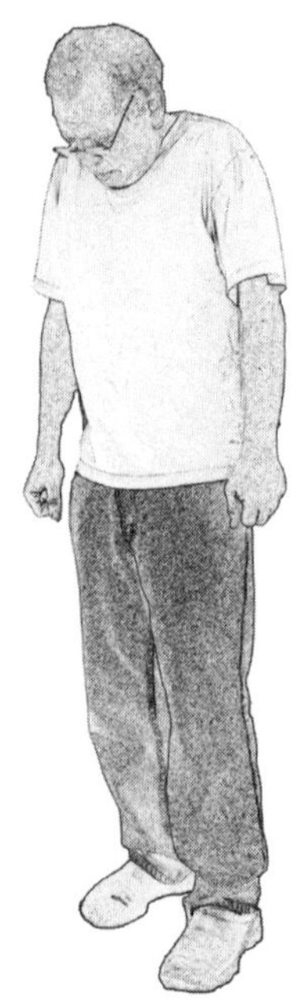

Exaggerated *default inner posture of shame* clarifying the pattern of muscle tension associated with chronic shame

Below are illustrations of the *default inner posture* of anger. The *default inner posture* is like an iceberg—99% of it is hidden. There are usually subtle (and sometimes not so subtle indications of it). In the figure on the left, we see how the man normally looks in his life. As the illustrations move toward the right, I show him exaggerating his *default inner posture* of anger. The last illustration in the series is the way this man would appear if he lost all control of himself and openly expressed the inner state he normally lives in. Except under exceptional circumstances, this all-out, disinhibited expression is rare to see. Representing his *default inner posture* in its most exaggerated form is meant to illustrate what this man carries around with him all of the time, but in a typically minimally expressed and hidden way.

## ***Default Inner Posture of Anger***

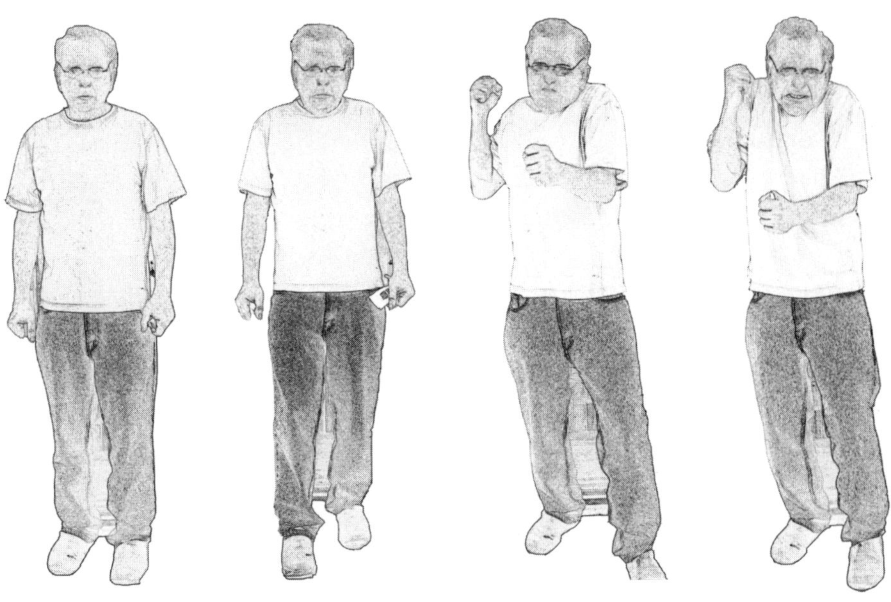

The normal appearance of the *default inner posture* of Anger illustrating the unexaggerated pattern of tension in the jaw, neck, shoulders, stomach, arms, and hands

Increasingly exaggerated expression of the *default inner posture* of anger clarifying the pattern of muscle tension associated with chronic anger

## Getting to know the *default inner posture* by having a dialogue with it

Because most people are not aware of their *default inner posture,* one helpful way of making it conscious and working with it is in a Gestalt therapy-inspired dialogue. In our clinic treating pelvic pain, I lead patients in a process in which they have a conversation with their tightened pelvis. This process is also appropriate for getting to know the *default inner posture.* The process goes something like this:

1. Feel a part of your body that is most tense.
2. Exaggerate this tension by making a caricature of it involving your entire body.
3. Note the emotion and attitude that would be most appropriate to describe this exaggerated posture. Typically the repertoire of emotions and attitudes related to the *default inner posture* are relatively few and include fear, anger, dread, disappointment, irritation, sorrow and grief and/or a combination of these emotions
4. Give a name to this default inner posture. For instance, if your name is Jim and you find the default inner posture within you is fear, you can call this 'Fearful Jim.'
5. You can now ask this part of you, while slightly exaggerating the *default inner posture* to stay connected to it, the following questions. Remember you are going to have to divide yourself into the questioner and the part of you who is being questioned. You'll get the most out of this if you are completely honest.
6. Ask this part of you, if this part of you is here, i.e., "Fearful Jim, are you there?"
7. Ask this part of you, how it feels that you are aware of it at this moment, e.g., "How do you feel, Fearful Jim, about me being aware of you?" Then put yourself in 'Fearful Jim's' shoes and do your best to respond as 'Fearful Jim.'
8. Ask this part of you, if it has any grievances against you and your treatment of it.
9. Ask this part of you, if there's anything you've done that hasn't been okay with it.

10. Ask this part of you, if there's anything you haven't done that it wishes you had done.
11. Tell this part of you, how you feel when you notice it inside you.
12. Ask this part of you, if it wants anything from you that you haven't given it, or if it hasn't wanted something that you have given it.
13. Ask this part of you, if it wants to say anything to you that has not been said already.
14. Ask yourself if there's anything you want to say that you haven't already said.

When we are aware of our *default inner posture* and are able to rest with it, it will tend to dissolve. The *default inner posture* is usually subtle and has been around in us for decades. Discerning this pattern of tension, re-identifying with it, and *inhabiting* it, giving it the space to exist, and resting with it make it easier to enter into a profoundly relaxed state.

# Chapter 7

## Understanding the role of attention training in *Paradoxical Relaxation*

## The key to becoming proficient at profound relaxation is being able to control your attention

Training attention to stay one pointed with minimal distraction is essential in reliably being able to calm down a nervous system that has a tendency toward anxiety. In contemporary western medicine, training attention is rarely discussed, except perhaps in relationship to the treatment of attention deficit disorder. Training attention as a central part of relaxation tends to be absent in the scientific conversation about relaxation and autonomic self-regulation. In this section, I discuss the training of attention as it relates to relaxation.

It took me many years to understand that
being able to control my attention was
essential in being able to profoundly relax

One of the cornerstones of *Paradoxical Relaxation* is the practice of maintaining seamless continual attention on a tensed part of the body as it relaxes. The task is to remain focused on tension as it releases without trying to make it relax and simultaneously to relinquish any unnecessary effort in doing so.

Attention is the joystick of the nervous system

At the beginning of the 20th century when airplanes first came on the scene, the lever that controlled an airplane's movement and direction was nicknamed the *joystick.* It is an eminently American nickname. Over the decades, the term *joystick* has been used to describe any lever-like switch for controlling, manipulating, guiding, or the like. As the age of computers matures and video games have become a huge part of the culture, the *joystick* is frequently used to control the action on the screen. The *joystick* is the control center.

Attention is the *joystick* of the nervous system. *If you are able to control your attention, generally speaking, you will be able to exercise remarkable control over your nervous system.* For example, if you direct your attention toward something upsetting, your nervous system will immediately respond with arousal and disturbance. If you direct your attention toward what is peaceful and uneventful, your nervous system will tend to be quiet. All things being equal, when you can control your attention, you most likely control the arousal levels of your nervous system.

If you want to 'pull someone's chain,' as the modern vernacular goes, you will say something that directs their attention to what arouses them. If you want to make someone feel good, you will direct their attention to something that is soothing to their nervous system. Optimists direct their attention to what is hopeful and not disturbing.

Pessimists direct their attention to what is negative—
optimists direct their attention to what is positive

Pessimists direct their attention to what is worrisome, hopeless, or disturbing. The cheerful person regularly pays attention to what is cheerful. The anxious person regularly pays attention to what is fearful. In the *glass half-full* analogy, the way you view the glass is all about what you do with your attention in relationship to it. As we see with Pollyanna, the only difference between seeing the glass half-full or half-empty is related to what aspect of reality or to which story you direct your attention.

You can think of the human organism as a 'response machine,' adjusting and responding to the different circumstances in the environment in order to survive. A central function of the nervous system is to respond with arousal to danger in the form of *fight, flight, or freeze.* When attention is not directed to anything fearful or disturbing, the parasympathetic branch of the autonomic nervous system is activated and restorative activities of tissue rejuvenation, healing and rest will dominate your experience. On the other hand, if you only pay attention to what you tell yourself is threatening, scary, ugly, and disturbing, the sympathetic branch of your nervous system is aroused and activated.

## One of the central skills of *Paradoxical Relaxation* is *controlling attention in order to rest it in sensation*

*The point in Paradoxical Relaxation is to rest attention in sensation and to turn attention away from the thoughts, interpretations, and distractions that pass through awareness.* In *Paradoxical Relaxation*, we practice receiving sensation directly, bypassing any judgements, or aversions, through which the sensation usually passes. Absent any attention to thought or distraction, the nervous system remains quiet. Controlling attention without strain is the key to the success of *Paradoxical Relaxation.*

## Brain activity and attention training

When you look at the hands of a carpenter, hands used to holding heavy hammers, saws, and lumber, you will notice that they invariably will be large and muscular. Similarly, when you examine the legs of a ballet dancer who daily practices leaping and dancing en pointe, you see legs that are strong and muscular. Your body and mind develop to support any activity that you do repetitively. Anything you practice, your body and mind will develop to help you practice more skillfully.

While it might seem unremarkable to observe the development of a carpenter's hand to more skillfully use construction tools, the scientific field of *neuroscience* has recently documented dramatic changes in the brain associated with repetitive activities. For instance, the part of the brain that is associated with the muscular activity of the fingers of the left hand of violinists shows dramatically more blood flow than the part of the brain associated with the activity of the fingers of the right hand, which simply holds the bow and isn't involved in the gymnastics of the fingers of the left hand. The same increased brain activity exists for the part of the brain associated with the fingers involved in piano playing.

There is a story of a prisoner of the Korean War, captive for a number of years, who practiced golf in his mind while confined to a cage-like jail cell. Every day during his captivity he would imagine the tiniest aspects of playing golf, from morning to evening. This included gripping the golf club, planting his feet, each swing, each club, long drives down the fairway, and the short putts on the green. Remarkably, when he was freed and came home, he was reputed to have scored under 100 in his very first golf game after having not physically touched a golf club for years. He had put in the necessary 'practice' hours; but in his case this practice was in meticulously visualizing playing golf rather than being on the golf course.

This is a striking example of using attention to visualize the practicing of a skill that you would think could only be practiced live and on the golf course. We see the profound power of controlled attention in this example.

This story is consistent with the recent discoveries about *neuroplasticity* in modern neuroscience, which have documented the development of the brain through simple mental rehearsal of some activity. Indeed, it appears you can practice the piano without even touching it and you will be strengthening the brain activity associated with playing the piano.

What is remarkable in the fledgling research emerging from neuroscience about attention is that paying attention is a peculiar kind of brain state, involving activation in parts of the brain that typically do not operate at the same time. Furthermore, those who have practiced paying attention for thousands of hours demonstrate a level of brain activity associated with paying attention that is unseen in the brains of those who have practiced no attention training.

## Mastering any skill means repetitively practicing it

By the time I had met Edmund Jacobson, I calculate that he had been practicing relaxation for approximately 25,000 hours. It has been said that those who are master musicians, tennis players, baseball pitchers, airplane pilots, machinists, and oil painters become masters of their art after they have put in 10,000 hours practicing what they do. This means 3 hours of practice per day for ten years. The point here is that just like a carpenter who has to have strong hands to hold a hammer all day (and has to have developed increased brain activity to support accurate hammering), so the brain develops to support the activity of sustained continuous attention.

Similarly, the development of competence in focusing attention requires many hours of practice to develop the brain activity associated with it. The goal in *Paradoxical Relaxation* is seamless, continuous, unbroken attention—no matter what your experience is during the relaxation. In other words, whether you are relaxing or not, whether you are feeling like you are getting anywhere or not, whether you are feeling happy or sad or good or bad, the goal in *Paradoxical Relaxation* is to maintain unwavering attention on tension as the tension releases, without trying to make the tension release.

In those with chronic anxiety, the nervous system and brain are used to being in an aroused state. If you tend to be anxious, you are good at practicing being anxious. Overcoming the tendency to live with an aroused nervous system means practicing what reduces this arousal.

## 40 hours of devoted *Paradoxical Relaxation* practice is usually necessary in order *begin* to calm down anxiety

One of the benefits of *Paradoxical Relaxation* is that you get better at it the more you do it. Over a lifetime, I believe it is the noblest of aspirations to put in the 10,000 hours necessary for mastery of this practice. Nevertheless, even 40 hours can *begin* to help you meaningfully calm down your anxiety. This means doing 1 hour of *Paradoxical Relaxation* every day for about 6 weeks.

## *Paradoxical Relaxation* is not taking a nap

When you take a nap, you let go of controlling your attention, you relax and let your attention go wherever it likes. And you usually fall asleep. In *Paradoxical Relaxation,* you are intentionally focusing your attention on the sensation of a particular part of your body. While you may drift in and out of sleep, you aspire to stay relaxed and focused.

The attention of the novice in *Paradoxical Relaxation* is usually undisciplined. Focusing this attention is not easy and the beginner quickly notices how easily his or her attention is distracted. Losing your focus usually occurs hundreds of times at the beginning of relaxation training. Beginners have to redirect attention away from thinking and back to the sensation which is the object of their focus.

*Paradoxical Relaxation,* in large part, is a special kind of attention training. Meditation has been described as a *royal battle* in which one fights to keep one's attention on the object of one's focus. As you get used to keeping attention focused, there is less struggle, and eventually, as you get to taste the fruits of controlled attention, the battle ends and the attention willingly and easily rests where you want it to rest.

When you have relaxed tension that you have chosen to focus on as much as it will easily relax, accept whatever sensation remains. Accepting tension, as I have emphasized throughout this book, often makes it go away. In *Paradoxical Relaxation,* I instruct patients to rest with a contracted sensation in their bodies on an ongoing basis without looking for an outcome, and to continue to focus continuously on the remaining sensation, doing their best to let go of evaluating or looking for benefit.

Paradoxical Relaxation is the moment
to moment assertion of your will

Practicing *Paradoxical Relaxation* and all of its subtle instructions of directing attention is a solitary act. You do it by yourself. No one is there with you other than the voice of the instructions when doing a recorded lesson. No one can monitor you. Choosing to follow the instructions discussed here and in other sections is a choice that must be reasserted over and over again, on a moment to moment basis.

*Paradoxical Relaxation* does not work if you are lazy. It works best if you sincerely and earnestly give yourself to carrying out its instructions. It works if you are willing to persevere with the myriad of times you fail to do the instructions perfectly. It works if you passionately commit yourself to unconditionally accepting yourself as you work with the instructions. It works if you are willing, if necessary, on a moment to moment basis, to reassert your will to accept tension and anxiety and all that such a practice entails. The continual assertion of your will refers to making a choice to focus your attention in a certain way.

## Focusing your attention inside your body

Each of us tends to have a default location in which we place our attention. Many people spend much of their lives with their attention externalized. They watch the news, they talk to and think about other people and tend to have to be 'doing something' in the world.

I came to understand this first hand during my days sketching and painting in cafes in San Francisco, one of my great joys in life. For many years, I spent hours every day doing this. Sketching someone without your attention being intrusive is something I had to learn how to do.

I noticed that there was a group of people who, no matter how considerately and unobtrusively I would glance over to see them, noticed my attention. Their attention was focused outward, scanning the environment and they were enormously sensitive to any attention being directed at them. Despite my skill at unobtrusively glancing over to catch the image that I sketched, I sometimes would have to give up sketching these people because even my deliberately unobtrusive observation made them uncomfortable. Their attention seemed to always be externalized, scanning their environment. My attempt to sketch them unnoticed could not escape their default externalized attention.

On the other end of the spectrum, there are people who tend to direct their attention inside themselves. I could look repeatedly at these people without them apparently noticing my attention. These people typically are lost in thought. There are many people who spend time 'up in their heads,' thinking, analyzing, figuring things out. There are professions that require this, such as computer programming, data analysis, and various kinds of research. For these people, their attention is focused on thinking. They are up in their heads. Their lives are lived mostly in their minds.

Other people whose attention is internalized may spend their time feeling the different sensations in their body. Artists, writers, and those interested in inner exploration typically focus their attention inside. Sometimes people whose attention is inside most of the time are hypochondriacs and are always scanning their physical experience for any signs of danger to their health. Some people have brought their attention inside to feel their emotions and examine their feelings and reactions. Psychotherapists often are in this group.

In *Paradoxical Relaxation,* students are asked to focus their attention on sensations inside the body. For people who have lived a life in which their attention has been primarily externalized, following the *Paradoxical Relaxation* instructions to direct their attention inside their body is a challenge.

## The repeated practice of being unconditional with yourself

When you direct your attention inside for extended periods of time, many emotions and reactions can arise in response to inner discomfort or anxiety. Your attitude toward these reactions can facilitate or interfere with your relaxation. One of the major lessons for those dealing with anxiety is learning to be unconditional with yourself whatever arises. By unconditional, I am referring to an attitude of, "I am going to be present with myself whatever I experience inside. Whether I am able to focus well, or am distracted, whether my symptoms reduce in this moment or not, whether I'm able to accept my tension or not, I will be here for myself without limitations or conditions. I will do whatever it takes, for as long as it takes, to help myself."

We usually treat ourselves the way our parents treated us. Few people had an ideal childhood in which parents had the time, energy, emotional balance, and wisdom to be unconditional with us. Most people want unconditional love, but few have ever experienced it beyond the fleeting moments of infancy. To be unconditional with yourself is to treat yourself the way you always wanted your loved ones to treat you.

Most of us have never completely devoted ourselves to our own care. *The relaxation protocol that I am describing requires time and patience.* I will often tell patients that while there are some general parameters of how long it takes for the symptoms to abate, when *Paradoxical Relaxation* works, it will take as long as it takes. People who practice relaxation with this unconditional attitude seem to do the best.

## For many, the world inside the body and mind is unknown territory

Making subtle distinctions about their internal sensations, particularly subtle levels of tension or relaxation, is often difficult for patients because it's not an activity that they've practiced. The tendency to avoid bringing attention inside the body is often, though not always, related to emotional pain from which someone has simply wanted to escape. The instruction asking students of *Paradoxical Relaxation* to keep attention focused on sensation, especially for those who've had little experience in introspection, at first is not easy, although it does get easier with practice.

If there are areas of discomfort in the body, there is a natural tendency to avoid and draw away from them. This tendency often occurs when there is constriction or discomfort related to anxiety or anxiety-related disorders. Your attention tends to want to focus anywhere but on the discomfort. We are programmed to pursue pleasure and avoid pain. The practice of *Paradoxical Relaxation* requires that you direct your attention back into your body even if it is initially uncomfortable to do so.

## Accepting tension is letting go of effort

*When you direct your attention to your sensation, which may include tension, with the goal to simply feel it and accept it, you are practicing the essence of Paradoxical Relaxation.* When I instruct you to feel the tension, I mean to let the tension be there without adding to or subtracting anything from it. When I say *rest with the tension,* I am instructing you to feel the tension and do your best to quiet yourself down while experiencing it. You are not trying to change the tension and there is no effort to be exerted to do so.

Imagine that you are lying directly on a wood floor without any pillows or blankets and you have not had any sleep in two days. You are completely exhausted and can hardly keep your eyes open. Now imagine that you are right on the edge of falling asleep. At that moment your muscles relax even though you are aware of the hardness of the wood.

You can consider your tension in the same way as you consider the wood floor. You are intimately connected with the tension as you are intimately in contact with the wood floor. In accepting tension, you are allowing yourself to rest deeply on the wood floor of your tension. *The difference between resting on the wood floor and resting with tension is that in resting with the tension, the tension itself will tend to relax as well, whereas the wood floor will not.* Your residual tension responds to your accepting attitude toward it.

In the practice of *Paradoxical Relaxation,* I offer you a strategy for dealing with the fear and aversion that can arise when you are relaxing with your discomfort. When attention is distracted, it should be returned remorselessly. Instead of being focused on the fear or aversion, I suggest you simply allow these feelings to be present in your experience. Coexist with them. Hang out with them. Allow them to be present without having to do anything about them. Feeling, resting, and allowing tension in this way is a practice of unconditionally accepting what is going on in your body in the moment.

## ***Paradoxical Relaxation* is the practice of being your own best friend**

Your tension responds to your unconditional acceptance in the same way that you respond to someone else's unconditional acceptance. Imagine you spend time with somebody who accepts you unconditionally. Imagine they communicate to you their commitment in the following way:

> *"I want to be present with you exactly as you are. I am not asking you to change in any way. While I may have preferences about how I might want you to be, I am committed to letting go of those preferences in favor of letting you be exactly the way you are. You may change from one moment to the next, and I am committed to being fully present with you on a moment to moment basis and feeling and accepting you however much you change. No matter what happens in this moment, I am determined to let you be as you are with an open and sincere heart."*

Most people would be very grateful to have a friend like this. When someone is present with us like this, we can relax. There is no danger of attack or judgment. The organism's emergency systems can rest, for there is no need to defend or protect oneself, no need for vigilance against danger. The attitude of such a friend is true support.

The tissues of your body respond to your unconditional acceptance of them in the same way as you respond to unconditional acceptance of others

Your tissues are imbued with your intelligence. These tissues have the same consciousness as you do. They recognize the presence of such an accepting attitude. When you regard yourself with patience and compassion, the tissues of your body know it. When you regard yourself negatively, the tissues also know it.

Most people are looking for relationships in which they are regarded in this unconditional way. In *Paradoxical Relaxation,* you are asked to have this kind of unconditional relationship with yourself, to be this kind of friend to yourself.

## Cultivating effortlessness

*Paradoxical Relaxation* is a practice of cultivating effortlessness. This means there is no strain, vigilance, bracing, protectiveness, doing, or action. Without training one's attention to stay one-pointed, the natural tendency of the mind is to think, that is, the natural tendency of the mind is to produce thoughts which are symbolic representations of reality in its different forms. This thinking generally keeps us from being effortless.

## Why letting your attention focus on thinking interferes with the experience of effortlessness

Why is it that thinking blocks effortlessness? The answer is that there is an instinctive and natural tendency *for the nervous system to respond to thoughts as if they were actually happening*, to take thoughts to be reality. The body responds, usually with some kind of tightening, as if the thoughts were real.

Jacobson did an experiment in which he measured the muscular response of different parts of the body when subjects imagined they were riding a bicycle. Remarkably, the parts of the body that slightly tightened were the hands and feet, which are normally involved in holding the handlebars and pedaling the pedals when riding a bicycle. The muscles involved in riding a bicycle were shown to be recruited in the imagined effort of bicycle riding.

Yogis are known to increase their heart rate up to 120 beats per minute by imagining they are running to catch a train that has left the station. We all intuitively know and have experienced a variety of thoughts producing strong physical reactions, as if the thoughts were real. Sexual thoughts can produce strong physical reactions involved in sexual arousal. Fearful thoughts can raise the heart rate and engage all of the other physiological activities involved in the survival response of fight, flight, freeze. Whenever we think, the response of the body is to tighten up and effort in a variety of ways.

REM (rapid eye movement) sleep is sleep specifically involved in dreaming. Dreaming is visual thinking. It is well known that REM sleep, while important in the sleep cycle, is often not restful sleep. Restful sleep comes from the cessation of dreaming and visual thinking. It is the absence of thoughts that produce effortlessness in sleep and thereby produce the most profound relaxation. As it is in sleep, so it is in the waking state. When attention rests in sensation and not in response to thinking, the most profound relaxation is possible.

To find the sensation in your body that you will focus on, your sincere effort is essential. Just like finding a street you have rarely been on or a passage in a book you read before, it takes effort to locate the sensation of tension. It isn't the gross, muscle tightening, sweat producing effort of moving a piano, but it is a very subtle effort of focusing attention that has a tiny bit of muscle tension attached to it. The focus of the eyes is always involved so when you feel your neck, for instance, your eyes tend to turn toward your neck. Once you have located the part of the body on which you are going to practice *Paradoxical Relaxation*, a certain kind of effort is necessary to keep attention in this area. This is especially true as other thoughts, desires, and particularly the instinct to avoid discomfort or pain.

As you become familiar with focusing your attention, less effort is necessary to stay focused and rest in sensation. You rest, relax, and reduce effort as you feel the sensation you have chosen to focus on. The point of *Paradoxical Relaxation* is to practice effortlessness at the deepest level, so that there is no sense of strain at all.

As you are more and more able to rest with tension, the effort required to stay focused diminishes and the line between you who is resting with the tension and the tension you are resting with becomes blurred. With more practice, you can merge into the tension which essentially dissolves it. This merger into the tension is the highest form of relaxation in which subject and object become one.

Presence of mind happens in the present moment. It implies having good judgment because your attention is fully here, attending to what needs attending to and not somewhere else, remote from the issue needing to be addressed. Unless you are here with whatever the problem is that you are confronting, your ability to address it is impaired. People get into accidents using cell phones because their attention is distracted from being here in this moment.

Presence of mind means that in this moment your attention is not distracted. It means that in considering what you are paying attention to, you are all there. It is a highly positive state, universally valued. To have presence of mind means that you can see clearly what you are focusing on, and being in this state implies that, being in full possession of your faculties and the facts of the situation, you know best what to do.

When you can focus on the *default inner posture,* when your mind is fully present with your tension, you can feel *that it is you doing the tensing.* Relaxing what has been chronically tense then becomes easy. It is easy because you have the presence of mind to feel the tension that, formerly, you have been tightening against automatically.

Re-identification with the *default inner posture* occurs when you have presence of mind in relationship to your residual tension. Patients have reported that when they have been able to focus their attention well, the primitiveness of the tension—how their tension has been protectively guarding out of fear—became clear to them.

When you have presence of mind you see all of this in a flash. It is not theoretical or intellectual. You experience it directly. It becomes clear over the noise of your anxiety that has come to feel normal (although never comfortable).

The ability to voluntarily reduce anxiety or relieve symptoms is a large event in someone's life and brings with it a level of satisfaction, self-confidence, and gratitude that usually does not come with the unbidden, uncontrolled reduction of symptoms. When anxiety and symptoms of anxiety-related disorders feel out of a person's control, the person often feels depressed or is left feeling helpless. Being able to reliably reduce anxiety and symptoms related to it using *Paradoxical Relaxation* may, in itself, be a better anti-anxiety strategy than any medication.

## The relationship between attention training and the reduction of anxiety

Sustained, focused attention is essential to reliable, profound relaxation in general and one's ability to reliably calm down anxiety in particular. When attention cannot be sustained long enough to permit you to become aware of the unconscious holding and guarding you are doing, this guarding tends to remain in place.

When students I have taught begin the first few days of *Paradoxical Relaxation* training, by far the most difficult obstacle that they encounter is the continuous and uncontrolled wandering of their attention. Dealing with distraction and the difficulty of focusing attention remains a theme throughout training in *Paradoxical Relaxation.*

How you come back from distraction is as important as maintaining seamless focus

## *Paradoxical Relaxation* and Aikido

Morihei Ueshiba, the father of the modern martial art of Aikido, was reputedly asked by one of his students how he remained so present and apparently unperturbed in the midst of combat. Whether apocryphal or not, he is reputed to have said that he did not consider himself exceptional at being continuously present in combat, but what he was really good at was 'coming back' from being distracted.

When people first begin *Paradoxical Relaxation* training, almost universally they report that their major frustration is staying focused. Their distress about being so often distracted by thoughts is usually allayed when they understand that the practice of *Paradoxical Relaxation* involves, like the skill of the Aikido master, getting good at 'coming back' from distraction. How you come back from distraction is as important as maintaining seamless focus.

## Mind-wandering during *Paradoxical Relaxation* is the most difficult obstacle to deal with at the beginning of training

*It is helpful for someone beginning Paradoxical Relaxation to know that when you begin practice, difficulty in focusing attention is the rule rather than the exception, normal rather than abnormal.* It is the nature of attention to wander. The tendency to be distracted and have attention flitting from one place to another is modifiable with practice, although this tendency will assert itself at different times, under a variety of circumstances. It is the rule and not the exception for the mind to wander *hugely* at the beginning of *Paradoxical Relaxation* training, despite all intentions to stay focused.

> It is helpful for someone beginning Paradoxical Relaxation to know that difficulty in focusing attention is the rule rather than the exception

Developing the ability to control attention and cultivate undistracted focus is not different than the development of any other skill. Whether it is learning to play the guitar, serve the ball in tennis, use new computer language, staying focused on what you are newly learning is a challenge because you are being asked to stay present with what feels uncomfortable and what you don't do well.

## Beginners at *Paradoxical Relaxation* often feel frustrated, irritated, or remorseful when they find they are distracted

Beginners often feel various degrees of frustration, irritation, and remorse when they find that their attention has wandered off into what they're having for lunch or some distressing thought about their symptoms. The frustration, irritation, and remorse come from an unrealistic expectation regarding the degree to which they will be able to keep their attention focused.

When beginning relaxation training, it helps to adjust to realistic expectations. As one progresses in this relaxation practice, students learn to return attention to the chosen sensation they are focusing on without any emotion or internal comment about being distracted. Coming right back from distraction without wasting a nanosecond reacting to it, is what it takes to get good at coming back.

There is no quick way to achieve this—practice, practice and more practice is the often unwelcome secret.

> Coming back well from distraction means cultivating patience and remorselessness with regard to your difficulty of maintaining focused attention

The reason that it is important to specifically address what it means to come back *well* from distraction is that the inner activity of staying focused in *Paradoxical Relaxation* is peculiar and often not experienced in most of life's situations. This peculiarity involves the fact that in *Paradoxical Relaxation* you are asked to do something that at first you fail at over and over again.

When you learn any new skill, you very rarely get it perfect in the beginning. Dealing with not being able to do something well, but practicing until you get good at it, despite your numerous failures, is critical in getting good at anything new you learn.

## Practicing shamelessness and remorselessness in *Paradoxical Relaxation*

When you first begin to do *Paradoxical Relaxation,* you are going to fail many more times than you succeed at controlling your attention. *One of the key requirements for successful attention training is learning how to deal with this continual failure and devoting yourself to following the instructions.* The question here is how to continue practicing the protocol with intention and energy despite the frequent experience of failing at carrying out the instructions.

In order to deal with this vital issue, students of *Paradoxical Relaxation* must cultivate remorselessness and shamelessness every time they lose focus. You cannot have your self-esteem or your hope of getting better tied to being able to flawlessly follow the relaxation instructions right from the start. *It is very important to understand that an absolutely necessary and unavoidable part of learning relaxation is managing the inherent, continued failure at staying focused, especially at the beginning of training.* This means that you consider it normal and proper that you fail at following the instructions over and over again. Every time you set the intention to focus your attention and then fail to do so, you must learn to regard this not as failure, but as a necessary part of learning the method.

In this way there must be no remorse when your attention wanders, no sense of, "Damn it, why can't I stay focused?," no feeling of frustration or anger or disappointment at having lost focus. There needs to be a sense of, "In losing my focus and then coming back, I'm doing it right and not doing it wrong."

> Practicing shamelessness and remorselessness about how often your attention gets distracted is particularly important if you tend to be a perfectionist

You can react with frustration when you say to yourself, "I'm going to do this" and then find yourself unable to do it. People who have had perfectionist parents and who have taken in that kind of perfectionism and made it their own, usually have little tolerance for not getting it right the first time, and certainly the third or fourth time. In *Paradoxical Relaxation,* you are regularly going to not get it right thousands of times. These little reactions to briefly losing control of your attention will add up and will undermine your practice. Managing these reactions is the key to success in *Paradoxical Relaxation.*

## Skillfully driving a car is a model for how to deal with the experience of regularly losing control of your attention

When you become a good driver, you necessarily have learned the skill of remorseless and shameless return of attention from distraction that I am discussing here. Driving a car necessarily means correcting tiny errors over and over again. In the moment of driving any car, anywhere, you do not simply set a course and then take your hands off of the wheel. When you veer ever so slightly off to the right, you immediately correct this 'error' by turning the wheel ever so slightly to the left. Inevitably, that correction is going to require another correction, which is then going to require another correction. From a certain point of view, driving is the management of the failure to keep your car going in an exactly perfect direction.

A good driver seamlessly and effortlessly makes these corrections without any remorse or shame or reactivity. These corrections to the direction that the car is going in, when someone is a good driver, are done effortlessly and without a thought that you are doing anything other than driving well. When good drivers occasionally veer over the line of the lane, they don't consider it a bad thing or judge themselves negatively; it is just one of the things that happens when you drive.

Being able to remorselessly return your attention from distraction is a variation on the practice of self-forgiveness

Being remorseless, shameless, and self-forgiving in doing *Paradoxical Relaxation* will be deeply tied-in to your ability to be self-forgiving about mistakes that you make in your life. Self-forgiveness in the face of making errors is not a small issue and one of the benefits of *Paradoxical Relaxation.* Practicing self-forgiveness during relaxation helps you to practice it in your life.

When we forgive ourselves we are most likely able to forgive others. When we are unforgiving toward ourselves, we tend to treat others similarly. The importance of shamelessness, self-forgiveness, and remorselessness during *Paradoxical Relaxation* cannot be emphasized enough.

In the largest picture, *Paradoxical Relaxation* is the devoted practice of accepting *what is.* We accept tension that does not let go because that is *what is* in that moment. Furthermore, we accept our resistance to accepting tension because that resistance is also *what is.* We accept pain and discomfort when that is present because that is *what is.* And despite our best efforts, especially at the beginning, the wandering of the attention is *what is.* To emotionally react to *what is*, especially with negativity, always adds an obstacle in quieting nervous arousal.

When you take seriously the practice of being shameless, remorseless, and self-forgiving when you are doing *Paradoxical Relaxation*, your ability to calm down in situations where you never thought it would be possible becomes possible. The kinds of situations you may never have thought you could relax in could include an emotional upset with someone, a health crisis, or a delicate negotiation.

## Practicing remorselessness while using *Paradoxical Relaxation* to go to sleep

One of the most rewarding places to practice remorseless return of attention is in dealing with sleep disturbance, including the inability to fall asleep and the inability to fall back asleep after you've woken up in the middle of the night. I will discuss sleep disturbance in more detail in the chapter on functional somatic disorders. Not being able to fall asleep is almost always related to being swept up in thoughts that assail you one after the other. When you practice remorseless return of attention from the distraction of thoughts, you may well find that your body will calm down, your thinking will slow, and more often than not you will fall off to sleep.

## Setting the intention to stay focused

To intend something means to make a decision to use all of your resources to bring it about. Setting an intention means you 'mean business'.

Setting an intention to stay focused separates the expert from the novice in *Paradoxical Relaxation.* The novice allows himself to lollygag, to allow his attention to float here and there as it naturally will do. Allowing attention to be uncontrolled means that you subject yourself to all of the various images and thoughts that cause the body to tighten up ever so slightly. The constant barrage of images provides an unending stream of stimuli that continue at some level or another to keep your nervous system aroused.

When you are able to rest your attention in sensation
and stop your thinking, the world goes away

To profoundly relax, it is necessary, in a certain sense, to remove yourself from the world by stepping out of the symbolic representation of the world created by your thoughts. My thoughts about the world or another as dangerous, uncaring or indifferent are examples of different symbolic representations of the world. The most profound relaxation is the relaxation is when thinking substantially slows down or stops. Without thought, the body is not responding to any symbolic image of the world and it can profoundly rest.

Setting the intention to focus on sensation is the first step. The mind naturally has many images that arise moment by moment—thousands of images a day. The intention to stay focused on sensation is necessary to gain control over the natural wandering of attention toward the myriad of thoughts that occur in the mind.

If you are genuinely interested in learning *Paradoxical Relaxation*, understanding the vital importance of controlling your attention is key. You can't be lazy in this department. You have to mean it. You have to be sincere and earnest about keeping your attention focused on sensation.

> The intention to stay focused must be reasserted thousands of times. Getting good at Paradoxical Relaxation means setting your intention to focus over and over again

Setting your intention to stay focused is using your will to control your attention moment by moment, over and over again. At first, setting your intention to stay focused on sensation will be frustrated over and over again by the wandering of your mind, so great patience is necessary.

In the training that I teach in *Paradoxical Relaxation*, I give patients a 50-lesson recorded course. The instructions that are reiterated every fifteen to thirty seconds, are all intended to remind the student to set the intention to stay focused. These lessons are particularly helpful in the beginning year or two of practice.

> When I can control my attention, I can relax easily even if I am anxious

## Dissolving anxiety by controlling attention

The revelation that I had to learn to control my attention in order to profoundly relax struck me deeply and continues to do so. It was a long time coming. I've discovered how utterly central the controlling of my attention is to my ability to quiet myself down. I've come to see through my own experience that when I can control my attention, I can relax easily even if I am anxious. When my attention is strong, I can enjoy unutterable inner quiet and joy. I have not been able to sneak around the requirement that I be in control of my attention. As I will discuss later, I learned that I must be remorseless about bringing my attention back into focus when I have been distracted.

When you are not frustrated by your mind's tendency to wander, it gets easier to focus your attention

Here is another paradox. When you do not get frustrated at the tendency for your mind to wander, the easier it gets to focus your attention. It does not work to fight the resistance to staying focused on a part of the body that is tight. There must be no force, frustration, or impatience. Desire for quicker results must be abandoned. The best attitude is "I am here forever with what I am focusing on and no matter what happens, I continue to return my attention when I find my minding wandering." This means postponing gratification. At first it requires having faith that you will reduce or stop your anxiety, tension, and related symptoms, even though you are being asked to give up wanting relief of anxiety, tension, and related symptoms in the moment.

## Grounding the ball: the process of breaking the cycle of negative thinking

When you play catch with somebody they throw the ball to you and you then throw the ball back, then repeat this over and over again. When you ground the ball, someone throws you the ball, you catch it, then put it down. You don't throw it back. You don't engage in interaction with the other ball thrower. In other words, you end the cycle of playing ball.

It has been said that the best strategy when being cross-examined by a lawyer is to 'ground the ball.' The lawyer asks you a question to trip you up and gain advantage by your answer. When you ground the ball in this context, your response is to say as little as possible and end the discussion. In *Paradoxical Relaxation,* the goal is to "ground the ball" when your attention gets caught in thinking. This means you don't engage in the thought that has distracted you, but instead return your focus to the place of tension you have chosen to feel.

## Directing attention back to sensation and away from verbal thoughts and mental pictures

It is essential to become practiced in focusing attention on sensation and not on a picture or thought of it. When you slip into a warm fragrant bath, you feel the warmth and support of the water and smell the fragrance in it. The bath experience is a sensory one and not an intellectual one.

The practice of Paradoxical Relaxation
focuses on sensation directly

During relaxation practice, when attention wanders to thinking, attention is repeatedly brought back to the experience of the sensation. *Getting good at Paradoxical Relaxation means getting good at keeping attention on sensation and quickly returning to sensation when the mind wanders into thinking.*

It is important to understand that correctly focusing on sensation in no way means that thoughts will not come into your awareness. Very often one can be absorbed in sensation while peripherally noticing thoughts coming in and out of awareness. This is absolutely fine. Becoming an adept in *Paradoxical Relaxation* means that you can stay focused on sensation as thoughts float in and out of awareness and not have your attention be pulled away by these thoughts.

## How can you tell the difference between paying attention to sensation as opposed to thinking?

When you rest attention in neutral sensation, your mind and body tend to quiet down. When you pay attention to sensation, you have to be in the present, neither going back to the past nor considering the future. Thoughts may flit in and out, but your attention rests on the sensations you are feeling. When attention shifts to thinking, some increase in tension and discomfort usually occurs.

The following metaphor can be useful in understanding how to keep attention focused on sensation rather than on thought. When walking down a crowded city sidewalk, many faces come toward you as they continue in the opposite direction. If you are clear about where you are going, you continue in your direction. While you may see many of the faces through the periphery of your vision, you don't stop to have conversations with these people. You simply go in your direction. I suggest that patients do the same thing with the thoughts that come into their awareness as they focus on feeling the sensations of tension. It is fine to be aware of thoughts peripherally as they come in and out of awareness, as long as you don't stop to engage with them.

## Continuing to feel the sensation in the area upon which you have chosen to focus

*You may notice that the tension subsides as you continue to feel and accept it.* You may feel this as a kind of easing. If tension in your shoulders is your focus, you may notice the shoulders drop slightly.

*This experience of relaxation tends to regularly occur when you accept tension.* You may find that as tension eases, a new and lower level of tension appears. It is like opening one door and walking down a hallway to discover another closed door. This second closed door is the natural reaction of the body to resist sudden precipitous change.

Understood in this way, the new lower level of tension is simply a way station along the road to complete relaxation. It is the body saying, "Okay, I can let go, but I can't let go all the way right now––so I'll let down a little." Tension is dynamic and changes and shifts regularly.

# Chapter 8

*Practice makes perfect*

## What you practice you get better at

The word practice has sources in French, Latin, and Greek. The French origin of the word practice is *practiser* which is to do something habitually. In contemporary language, to practice simply means to do something over and over again. This applies from the practice of *Paradoxical Relaxation* to making the cabinets for Steinway pianos.

> *"You can teach somebody how to do a job, but only time makes them better. The longer they do it, the better they get at it."*
>
> \- *Craftsman at Steinway piano factory*

As a rule, whatever you practice you get better at. What I have discovered in my relaxation practice is that if I don't stay on top of the tendency for my attention to flit around, the quality of my relaxation suffers. If I miss doing relaxation for a day, my life suffers. Simple as that. And thus I've realized that I can't afford to not practice the method I describe here in this book.

## There is no substitute for practice

Becoming competent in *Paradoxical Relaxation* requires many hours of practice and then daily practice after that. In our pelvic pain clinics, we give our patients a 50 lesson course that needs to be done consistently over a period of a year and a half once they leave the clinic. The regular daily practice is what makes it effective. This practice is essential for anyone who wishes to use *Paradoxical Relaxation* to reduce anxiety.

It has been said that in real estate the three most important factors are: Location, location, location. In a parallel aphorism, it has been said that there are three rules for managing wealth: Don't lose it, don't lose it, don't lose it.

*In the same way, there are three rules to learning Paradoxical Relaxation: Practice, practice, practice.* The only way I have been able to improve my ability to quiet down my body and mind is to practice controlling my attention, accepting tension, letting go of my preferences and releasing my aversion to my own demons and fearful thoughts.

Relaxation requires that I practice not resisting what is uncomfortable or painful, that I practice not arguing with reality, that I practice accepting and resting with whatever the sensation is and that I practice letting go of the outcome.

## What does it mean to *have a practice*?

As I get older and the inevitable difficulties, losses, and tragedies occur to myself and people around me, it is clear to me that people who have practiced relaxation, calming down their nervous system, and returning from their agitation to peace, fare far better in life, especially as life gets more difficult. Those who *have a practice* are generally those who practice daily some form of relaxation training or meditation.

The hardest part of exercise is showing up at the gym—at first the hardest part of Paradoxical Relaxation is showing up to do a relaxation session

Those of us who are committed to doing physical exercise in the midst of busy lives know that the hardest part of maintaining a physical exercise regimen is getting oneself to the place where we exercise. If my agreement with myself is that all I have to do is to show up there, invariably the exercise I came to do gets done. Everything else is easy. At first, the hardest part of becoming skilled in *Paradoxical Relaxation* is regularly showing up to do it.

Repetition is the mother of retention

The fragile ability to rest below the symptom threshold for many people who suffer with anxiety is the reason why it is necessary to repetitively reduce nervous system arousal. This must be done over and over again. Learning to relax, if you are normally anxious, from the conditioned level of anxiety and arousal that you normally inhabit, to the place of quiet and of peace. Persistent, non-discouraged practice of 'resetting' the speed of the nervous system to a non-anxious level gets the body and mind used to being in such a quiet state.

In my experience, you will be disappointed if you have the belief that, after only a few successful relaxation sessions in which anxiety and related symptoms quiet down, you should be able to stop your conditioned and upregulated nervous system. This disappointment is not helpful and it is based on ignorance about the extent of practice required to calm down a chronically anxious and aroused nervous system.

## *Getting real* about what is possible in the short term and long term

At first, if you are suffering from anxiety, it is best to focus on reducing anxiety rather than thinking you should immediately eliminate it. Relaxation is not about *hitting a home run* and having things change quickly and permanently. Having realistic goals is important or you will be disappointed. This is why I emphasize the necessity of repetition to again restore balance and rest to the nervous system and softness to the tissue.

## How my relaxation practice helped me survive my brother's death

Years ago, my older brother became ill with an aggressive recurrence of leukemia. The 8 months that passed between the beginning of the recurrence of his illness and his death was a very difficult time for me. I was his bone marrow donor for his failed bone marrow transplant. I was also one of his major supports. Those 8 months occurred through a cold winter in New York, far away from the comfort and support of my California home. Many things went wrong during my brother's illness; ultimately, the bone marrow transplant didn't work and my brother died.

What is clear to me now is how important my relaxation practice was for me in keeping some perspective and balance. In the midst of sorrow, anxiety, agitation, and isolation, living mostly in a hospital room with a surgical mask and gown in a cancer hospital to support my brother, I did relaxation. While my understanding of relaxation was no where then what it is now, I practiced relaxation every day. It was often not easy. In the midst of this great stress, I was able to inwardly rest and keep some semblance of balance.

It is difficult to dig the well when the house is on fire

It is best to have a well dug before you need the water in it to put out a fire. Digging the well when the house is on fire is not the easiest thing to do. This aphorism illustrates a strong message about the obvious importance of preparation. The same idea is conveyed by saying that it is better to study for a test before the day of the test, it is better to have practiced a musical piece before you perform it, and it is better to have practiced tennis before you enter into a tennis tournament.

In dealing with the crisis of my brother's illness and death, which made calming down my very agitated nervous system so difficult, I depended on the relaxation practice I had done when there was no crisis going on in my life, when the house wasn't on fire. I had dug a rudimentary well before the house caught fire.

## Having a practice to calm nervous arousal and enter into a state of equanimity is especially important as you face the inevitable difficulties of aging or suffer from the physical symptoms of anxiety-related disorders

Recently I spoke to a friend whose 18 year old son was leaving home and who was dealing with *empty nest syndrome.* My friend has been practicing meditation for many years and is able to quiet down her mind and body with unusual skill. She told me that while her son's departure from home and her changing role as a mother had its moments of discomfort, her meditation practice returns her to a place inside of deep relaxation where she is happy. My friend seemed quiet and peaceful about the possibilities of how she was going to furnish her *empty nest.*

## A perspective on how to view misgivings about taking the time that is necessary to do relaxation

You have to devote time and energy for any relationship in your life to flourish. It is hard to imagine having a meaningful relationship when you make no time for it. It is not possible to become skillful with *Paradoxical Relaxation* unless you devote time to it. Sometimes patients have symptoms of anxiety or related disorders that require them to devote what they feel is an inordinate amount of time to calming themselves down.

It is not uncommon for people with anxiety and anxiety-related disorders to fret and feel guilty about having to take so much time in taking care of themselves. If you practice *Paradoxical Relaxation,* you will need to take a good hour out of your day to do relaxation, plus additional time for other potential modalities, including self-treatment physical therapy and stretching, depending upon whether you have physical symptoms.

During certain times when I suffered from pelvic pain, I remember feeling that aside from the most basic things in my life, I was having to devote almost *all* of my time to relaxation, physical therapy self-treatment, and working with my mind to get through the day. I felt badly about this. Like many people who deal with similar conditions, I had no one to talk to about this. I felt badly that I was a party pooper and didn't feel like, or wasn't capable of, managing a social engagement.

I felt badly about deciding to withdraw from many activities in my life because of my anxiety and related symptoms. These activities included going out to dinner or planning a trip with family or friends. I avoided going back to Canada where I am from because of the long plane ride and stress of traveling. At times, when something happened in the family, such as a relative dying or someone in my family having a big event, I felt I just couldn't manage the trip. One time, my aunt was angry with me for not coming back to my uncle's funeral and I felt terrible, but I knew I just couldn't tolerate the stress and pain of the trip. I felt that my symptoms would be materially worsened if I went.

## The airlines know that in an airplane emergency, you put your own oxygen mask on first before you put on the mask of your children: it is a kindness to everyone in your life to take care of your anxiety

There is a very clear reason why the airlines tell you to put on your own oxygen mask before you put on the oxygen mask of your children. If you are gasping for breath, you will be far less effective in concentrating on helping anyone else. Your panic in not having taken care of yourself will spill over to those you are trying to help. It just doesn't work to not take care of your own need for oxygen when you are responsible for the oxygen needs of others.

## If you are the source of water, no one wants your well to go dry

The same concept about putting on your oxygen mask first applies to not letting your well go dry if you are the source of water for those you love. This is particularly true for children and family members who rely on you in various ways. I have often told patients that the biggest gift you can give those who love you and depend on you in various ways is to take care of yourself, and to get better.

To put this in perspective, think of the gift it would have been for you if your mother or father would have devoted time each day to their own self-care and would have emerged from this time feeling happier, more peaceful, more emotionally available and more giving. Few of us would have resented their taking the time to care for themselves. On the contrary, we would have wanted them to take care of themselves and we would have gladly given up that time to them.

## The best thing you can do to take care of those whom you love is to take care of yourself

Most people I have treated with anxiety and anxiety-related disorders have been conscientious to a fault in terms of fulfilling obligations and taking care of those depending on them. The obstacle to this giving has been the significant and sometimes disabling distress of their own anxiety or anxiety-related disorder. Typically, however, when their inner distress calmed down, taking care of others who depend on them is easy and often filled with joy.

> If you want to stop feeling guilty about how much time you spend in taking care of yourself, you must find a way to forgive yourself for your condition

If it is true that the biggest gift you can offer others in your life is to take care of yourself and bring peace into your own life, then it becomes clear that self-judgments about your condition make no sense. When I realized that the best thing I could do for my loved ones and for my world was to take care of myself, I had to find a way to forgive myself for having pelvic pain. And I was able to do this. I stopped taking my condition personally. I knew that if I had been given a choice about having pelvic pain or not, I would never have chosen it. I learned not to take the fact that I had it personally, as if I had made some terrible mistake or committed some sin.

I gave up the idea—which is not an uncommon idea among those with anxiety and anxiety-related disorders—that somehow I brought it on myself or that I was being punished for something. I saw that both ideas were absurd. I saw that I was doing the best I knew how to do in my life when I started having pelvic pain and that if I would have known a way to stop my symptoms back then, I certainly would have stopped them.

Viewing anxiety as some kind of punishment is a story some anxious people tell themselves in order to try to find some rhyme or reason why they are anxious or have anxiety-related physical symptoms. Such thinking, in my mind, is an attempt to get rid of the idea that you have no control over your life or anxiety by holding on to this irrational idea of cause and effect even if the cost of such an idea is debilitating and makes you more anxious. Very often the negative stories some anxious people tell themselves about why they are suffering with anxiety serve no function other than to create more suffering in their lives.

I found in times when I had to spend hours and hours, sometimes most of my discretionary time taking care of myself, I coached myself by saying that I wouldn't always have to do this. At the time I had to devote an inordinate amount of time to my self-care. I sometimes thought that if I had a sick child, I would not begrudge or feel badly about devoting all of my time to my child. I would tell myself that *I* was my sick child at that particular moment and that it was out of love and care for myself (and ultimately all those who loved me) to accept that, for now, I had to devote this amount of time to myself.

There are different kinds of selfishness in my mind. There is selfishness that is small and focuses narrowly on your own pleasures and needs. And then there is selfishness, that when pursued, helps everyone. In my view, taking care of my own well being is the best way I can take care of the world. The happy, peaceful person in the world is a light for everyone.

# Chapter 9

## Catastrophic thinking and *Paradoxical Relaxation*

## Catastrophic thinking projects catastrophe or calamity into the future and is gasoline on the fire of anxiety and anxiety-related disorders

Linda and Jim had been married for 6 years and had never been apart for a night. Jim had a strong tendency toward anxiety and was uncomfortable being alone without the company of his wife for any period of time let alone a whole night. At the 6 year mark, Linda was asked to speak at a conference on the other side of the country from where they lived at a time when Jim was unable to take off from work. Speaking at the conference would mean a lot to Linda and would also mean that Linda would have to be away for 4 days. Normally Jim accompanied Linda to these kinds of events, but because he couldn't go, at Linda's insistence, Jim agreed for Linda to go to this conference by herself even though he was quite anxious about being apart from her.

Linda's trip went quite well. Jim and Linda spoke several times a day and Jim felt good that he was able to manage being apart from Linda for the few days she was gone. Jim was at work on the day Linda was supposed to come home and was a little anxious about her flying. He expected to hear from her before she boarded the plane and his anxiety ramped up when he did not. He became increasingly anxious when the plane had arrived and he did not hear from her. He began to panic a half hour after the plane had arrived.

Jim had a tendency to think catastrophically and his catastrophic thinking began in earnest after he had not heard from her. His mind went wild and he became panicked. Had she been in a car accident and been killed on her way to the airport? Was she kidnapped, raped, murdered? Had she met another man and left him? Did she have a heart attack and was in the intensive care unit? Did she take the wrong plane? Did something bad that he couldn't even imagine happen?

An hour after she was supposed to have arrived, Jim began calling the police departments and hospitals in the city Linda had visited. He frantically called Linda's family and her close friend to see if they had heard from her. They hadn't. Jim couldn't figure it out. His mouth went dry, his palms became sweaty, he felt an old familiar pain in his stomach and he felt dizzy as he felt his heart pound and then skip beats. He became worried that he was having a heart attack. He began imagining his own death, the death of his wife, the terrifying prospect of being alone without Linda and other catastrophic outcomes. And all of these stories of catastrophe were triggered by Jim not hearing from Linda before she was supposed to have left the airport and a little after she was supposed to have arrived.

Then Jim thought that maybe she had left a message for him at home so he called home. There was a message on his home phone that stopped the nightmare he found himself in. Linda's cell phone had gone dead and Linda was calling from the airport from a pay phone telling Jim that she had never learned his cell phone number by heart because it was always programmed into her cell phone which was then not working. Jim had never considered that Linda would leave a message on the home number because she always called him on his cell phone. And like many times in his life, he felt huge relief as well as shame at the story he concocted that made his nervous system go crazy. Such a scenario of catastrophic thinking then followed by relief and feeling foolish were an almost daily occurrence for Jim.

When you have a tendency toward catastrophic thinking, you regularly make up stories that at a certain level you are convinced are true. You believe that the worst has already happened. Catastrophic thinking whips up a panic in the body. It assumes, with certainty, that the worst has happened.

In the moment of catastrophic thinking, there is no doubt that the catastrophic thought has occurred. The catastrophic thought feels real and to not pay attention to it means that you are going to be surprised by it later if you put it out of your mind now. Catastrophic thinking is aimed at protecting you from being unprepared for bad things happening. In the story above, Jim was thinking catastrophically to protect himself from being surprised by the worst thing happening. His catastrophic thinking, as with all catastrophic thinking, consisted of stories he made up that came from a primitive part of his mind that wanted to protect him, but ultimately routinely made his life miserable.

Uncontrolled fearful and catastrophic thinking plays a seminal role in ongoing states of anxiety and is part of a self-feeding cycle in anxiety and anxiety-related functional disorders. If you are anxious or have an anxiety-related physical condition and you don't gain control over your tendency to think negatively and catastrophically, your suffering will probably continue.

Catastrophic thinking can revolve around your life with friends, family, work, health, safety, economic security, whether you are going to get in trouble with the law, among many other subjects. It includes thoughts like, "I'll always feel lonely, my life is a waste, I'll never experience real intimacy, I'll never find happiness, this pain is probably cancer or the precursor of a heart attack, my boss' unfriendliness today means I'll be fired and eventually homeless, this registered letter probably means someone is going to sue me..." and on and on.

When there is a physical condition associated with anxiety, catastrophic thinking can often strongly exacerbate the symptoms. We discussed this extensively in our book on pelvic pain, *A Headache in the Pelvis*. Tension feeds anxiety, which feeds any pain that might be part of the condition, which feeds protective guarding, which continues to go around and around. Discomfort or pain causes you to tighten the muscles to protect against the ongoing experience of anxiety and discomfort, which instead of helping the anxiety and discomfort, actually increases them. This protective guarding triggers catastrophic thinking and more anxiety.

Both a peaceful mind and a troubled mind ultimately do not depend on what happens to you but on how you view what happens to you

When your mind is peaceful, your thoughts are peaceful. When your mind is troubled, your thoughts usually engender anxiety and suffering. Effectively managing negative and dysfunctional thinking makes the major difference between being able to calm down an aroused nervous system or not.

Said another way, suffering does not come from the circumstances of our lives, but from our viewpoint toward these circumstances. Our viewpoint comes in the form of thoughts. This is not a new idea. This enduring insight has been expressed in schools of modern psychology over and over again in ancient wisdom traditions.

In the *Bible*, there is a saying in Proverbs that, 'As a man thinks, so he is.' In the *Dhammapada* it is stated that, 'Our thoughts create our world—we are what we think—all that we are arises with our thoughts—with our thoughts we make the world.'

So anxiety and an aroused nervous system are intimately connected with your thoughts. Your thoughts represent the world to you. If your thoughts represent your life as dangerous you become anxious. If you see life as safe and supportive and loving, there is no anxiety. Let's remember that anxiety is a protective response. It is a way an organism mobilizes itself to stay alive in the face of threats to survival.

## The aim of *Paradoxical Relaxation* and cognitive therapy is the same

When you do *Paradoxical Relaxation,* you rest your attention in sensation. Your job is to not engage in thinking. *Paradoxical Relaxation is the practice of resting attention outside of thinking.* When the tension rests outside of thinking, the body does not have to respond to the world or a representation of the world. This is why non-REM sleep is the most restful sleep; the body is not responding to any world created in the dream state. Dreaming is just a certain kind of thinking that goes on during sleep.

When we do *Paradoxical Relaxation,* we do not evaluate the content of our thoughts. We don't analyze whether a catastrophic thought is true or not. Our job, no matter what the thought is, is to bring our attention back to sensation and ignore having any relationship to the thought. In a way, this is like cleaning out an attic full of old letters without reading any of them. They all go.

While *Paradoxical Relaxation* is the practice of releasing negative and catastrophic thoughts without examining them, what has come to be known in conventional psychology as Cognitive Therapy, is the practice of releasing negative and catastrophic thoughts by examining them and evaluating their validity. The clear aim of both is in helping to free you from the grip of catastrophic thinking.

The very act of reducing nervous system arousal makes it easier to recognize cognitive distortions and let them go

This idea is included in the conventional wisdom that things will look better in the morning after a good night's sleep. This idea reflects the common experience that when you are tired, upset, and nervous, you can't see things the way you can when you are rested and calm.

The therapy of *Paradoxical Relaxation* that allows you to come into peace and equanimity is a most powerful cognitive therapy as well. Both conventional cognitive therapy and *Paradoxical Relaxation* have the aim of rescuing the nervous system from the grip of negative and catastrophic thinking. Conventional cognitive therapy focuses on the content of the dysfunctional thinking to disarm its ability to disturb the nervous system. *Paradoxical Relaxation* simply removes attention from all thinking, rests it in sensation and in so doing makes you much better able to just see the distortion of the negative thinking on its face and dismiss it out of hand.

## Cognitive therapy that assists *Paradoxical Relaxation*: evaluating the validity of negative thoughts

In the midst of our lives, we obviously cannot stay away from thinking in the way that we do during the relaxation session. Negative and catastrophic thinking is much more likely to affect us during our waking and active hours. It is important in lowering the general level of nervous arousal to identify specific troublesome thoughts that can ignite our nervous system. As I discuss in detail in the following section on anxiety, the work of Byron Katie is the most easily accessible in helping one deal with these thoughts.

## Disarming negative and catastrophic thinking is neither simple nor quick but you can get good at it

It takes a long time to extricate yourself from a routine tendency to catastrophize, to jump to the worst case scenario given little or no evidence of the catastrophe. It is helpful to have great patience with yourself in dealing with catastrophic thinking. Once you recognize the negative consequences of thinking catastrophically and see the value of stopping catastrophic thinking, berating or judging yourself for not being able to simply stop this tendency to catastrophize serves no purpose. Thinking that you can quickly stop catastrophizing after a lifetime of doing it is like one day picking up the violin and being upset that you can't play like the masters.

Being able to stop thinking catastrophically, if you do so on a regular basis, is not simple. Catastrophic thinking is typically a way your subconscious conditioning tries to keep us safe Early conditioning, that is usually deeply ingrained, has us believe that jumping to catastrophic conclusions protects us from pain and vulnerability. Catastrophic thinking, as I have discussed elsewhere, is a defense against being surprised by what you imagine will hurt you. As crazy as it may appear, its purpose at root, from the point of view of your conditioning, is to help you survive.

## Witnessing a catastrophic thought

It is a big step to just be able to witness that you are having a catastrophic thought and that the catastrophic thought is just a thought, a story about your life that you made up. Witnessing the catastrophic thought means stepping back from it and seeing it as a *story* about the future and not necessarily the *reality* about the future. In fact, for most people, their catastrophic thoughts almost never come true.

Most people who are caught in catastrophic thinking don't even know it. These people are lost in the thought and there is little ability to stand back and say, "I'm catastrophizing again." There is little ability to let the thought be an object in awareness. They make no distinction between the thought and reality. They believe their thought is real. To be able to witness the thought is the very necessary first step in being able to live a life in which your mind does regularly catastrophize and drive you crazy. It is the first step in harnessing your mind as your servant and not your tyrant.

Even if you notice the catastrophic thought, it isn't helpful to think that doing a simple exercise is immediately going to get rid of it. When someone thinks this way, he often also thinks that if the catastrophic thought continues to linger despite his initial efforts, that he will never be free of catastrophic thinking. As you learn to deal more effectively with catastrophic thinking, you learn not to measure your progress by whether you can simply disappear the thought with an exercise but by how long it took you to release yourself from it.

If you are suffering with a catastrophic thought, rather than wanting it to just go away, first *notice how long it takes for you to notice the thought you are stuck in.* It is common to get so merged in the thought that it takes a long time to even notice that you're doing the same old catastophizing thing again. Often people suffering with anxiety don't know that their anxiety is coming from a thought because that thought is so vivid and real and they have never stood back to witness it.

There are things that happen in your life and then there is your story about the things that happen - the quality of your life reflects your story

There are all the events that happen in your life and then there is your particular story or 'spin' on these events. *Most people don't know that the quality of their lives reflects the stories they tell themselves about their lives.* This is a key and transformative insight. The problem with dysfunctional and catastrophic thinking is that the thought is so vivid you can't distinguish the difference between thought and reality. The task in dealing with catastrophic and dysfunctional thinking is to make this distinction to your nervous system.

Your body responds to the story you tell yourself as if your story were reality

When you deal with chronic anxiety or anxiety-related disorders, this confusion between catastrophic thinking and reality usually perpetuates the anxiety and the physical disorders related to it.

Catastrophic and dysfunctional thinking is usually about defending yourself from disappointment

When you examine your deepest motivation in jumping to a catastrophic conclusion, you will probably find that the catastrophic story is about protecting yourself from disappointment. *In a peculiar and irrational way, many anxious people believe they gain some control over their situation by thinking they are not going to get hit, or at least surprised, by bad things happening, if they think the worst.* Disappointment is an underrated human suffering and we human beings appear to exert great efforts to protect ourselves from disappointment. And the mind goes to great lengths to defend against it.

## Waking up our nervous system to distinguish thought from reality

It is helpful to notice the time at which the catastrophic thought starts and what the duration of the thought is (minutes, hours, days) before it peters out. Being able to be a witness to this process going on inside you is an important step because what you are doing is disidentifying with the thought. You are saying, "This is a thought that is coming up in me and disturbing me. Let me see how long it is going to stick around." This is another act of standing back and seeing the thought as a thought and not necessarily reality.

My description of this process is rarely sufficient to become proficient at it. Working with Byron Katie directly or someone trained in the method is much more helpful than just reading about the method. Information specifically about this cognitive therapy work can be found at www.thework.com website.

Practicing *Paradoxical Relaxation* in the middle of catastrophic thinking is a milestone. What it means is that you've decided to practice taking your attention away from the negative thought in the face of the conditioning that most people have when they think catastrophically. This conditioning typically translates into the thought: "You don't want to be surprised by taking your attention off the catastrophic thought because if you take your attention off of it, you are going to get negatively surprised, hurt, or disappointed."

Practicing *Paradoxical Relaxation* in a devoted way means practicing taking your attention away from the catastrophic thought and resting it in sensation. This represents another level in the development of your ability to not be a victim to your catastrophic thinking. Catastrophic and negative thinking are like flypaper to the anxious person; as soon as you get stuck on them, it is very hard to get them off of you.

Learning to see the catastrophic thought as words and pictures in your mind can help wake you up to the fact that the thought is a thought and does not necessarily reflect reality

## A structure to evaluate the validity of catastrophic thinking

### Step One: Finding the core thought

What can help disarm catastrophic thinking involves identifying the core thought that your fear and anxiety rest on. Typically, the chronically anxious person lives in a frightened world of negative thoughts that is rarely shared with anyone. Each negative thought is taken to be real by the body as it contracts against the scary world created by the thought. These scary thoughts inflame the anxiety or anxiety-related disorders.

Formulating a disturbing thought as a clear statement and not a question is helpful when working with your catastrophic thinking

A negative thought inventory is a list of your most common catastrophic thoughts that fuel much suffering in anxiety and anxiety-related disorders. Listing the negative or catastrophic thoughts as clear statements and stating them as if they are a certainty frames them in the way in which the body hears them. This reformulation makes the sting of these thoughts easier to identify and deal with when their validity is questioned by this process.

The cognitive therapy process works best with core thoughts that are simple declaratory statements. It is useful to write down these thoughts in the form of sentences. Instead of the thought, "Will I lose my job and be destitute?" the reformulation of the thought turns out to read, "I will lose my job and be destitute."

It is also useful to take the catastrophic thoughts that appear tentative and make them definitive. The thought, "Maybe I am going to lose my job and be destitute," then becomes, "I am going to lose my job and be destitute."

**Step Two: Face the core thought with openness and curiosity**

Like anxiety, the negative thoughts are not your enemy. They come from a frightened person's struggle to protect him or herself. The thought of consciously facing one's negative thinking can appear daunting and depressing. This approach, however, in clearly formulating the core negative thoughts and then examining their validity, usually lightens their impact. In learning to face and evaluate the validity of the negative thinking, it is often possible to soften or neutralize this kind of thinking. It is best to face negative thinking with curiosity and an interest in seeing whether the thoughts are true.

**How to evaluate the validity of the core thought from your body's reaction to it**

It is sometimes useful to experiment with bringing attention to the feeling in your chest and heart area. Feel the breath and the sensation in your chest as the air comes in and out. With your eyes closed and your attention on your heart and chest area, say your name and feel the feeling in the chest. For example you might say, "My name is John" or, "My name is Lindsey" and then you feel the sensation in your chest of truthfully saying your name.

Now keep your attention in your chest area and finish the sentence, "My name is________," using a false name. If your name is John, see how it feels in your chest to say that your name is Walter or Dennis. You will probably feel a little tightening or strangeness in your chest. Experiment with feeling your chest as you say your true occupation (e.g., I am an engineer) and then notice the feeling in your chest when you don't tell the truth (e.g., I am a baker or kindergarten teacher).

The point of this exercise is to feel your body's reaction to what is true and what is not true. The body can help you address the validity of your negative thoughts. Refer to the sensation in your body as you address the questions below.

**Examining the validity of the core thought**

After you have identified the core thought, ask the following questions to yourself about the thought. Feel the area in and around your chest and respond to the questions from this area. In other words, your answers should agree with the feeling in your chest area.

Question your core thought as follows:

1. Is this black or white, all or nothing thinking?
2. Is this thinking magnifying the negative and minimizing the positive?
3. Is there any action that you need to take about what you are catastrophizing about? Have you taken this action? Is there anything other than suffering that this thought offers?
4. Does this thinking discount the positive or hopeful?
5. Is this thinking generalizing one negative experience to your whole life?
6. Is this thinking blaming yourself for what you aren't responsible or aren't entirely responsible for?
7. What is the evidence I have for this core thought?
8. Using this evidence, can I say for sure that this thought is true?
9. What happens physically and emotionally inside me when I believe that this thought is true?
10. What has been the effect of this thought or this kind of thought on my life in the past?

11. What would happen to my life if I simply were incapable of thinking this thought or this kind of thought?
12. What is the opposite kind of thought to this one?

I ask patients to notice the effect of this questioning on their mood and the general impact that this thought has upon them. Catastrophic and negative thinking has usually been practiced for a long time. Doing this questioning process needs to be done often at the very moment that these kind of thoughts arise. It is possible for this process to help reduce the level of suffering that attends anxiety.

## Some thoughts about dealing with catastrophic and dysfunctional thinking

Dealing with our thoughts that needlessly cause us suffering is a lifelong process and a core curriculum for any thoughtful person interested in being happy. When you are in an *anxiety state*, the effect of your thinking is magnified. People who have a tendency toward anxiety should understand that without paying attention to the effect of their thoughts on their life, that they will likely be routinely victimized by their negative thoughts and tendency to catastrophize.

Here are some guide posts on the way to gaining control of negative, catastrophic and dysfunction thinking.

- It is essential to remember that there is a difference between what goes on in your life and your story about it
- A story is just a thought; your story about things may often not be true
- Your negative story or thought about the future may or may not describe what will happen in the future
- You don't have to take your thoughts personally
- You can't always believe what you think
- While catastrophic thoughts are almost always wrong, understand that the body responds to thoughts, right or wrong, as reality
- People usually grow when many times, they go through the cycle of having catastrophic thoughts, becoming anxious, and experiencing

the resolution of the catastrophic thinking. As you go through the cycle of catastrophic thinking resolving itself enough times to see the exaggeration and incorrectness of this thinking, you can begin to laugh at yourself and your thinking. Going through this cycle enough can help you not take your catastrophic thinking so seriously as it continues to occur.

- Freeing yourself from your catastrophic thoughts and your tendency to fret, worry, and always imagine the worst is a lifelong task. Such freedom will help you with many things that trouble you in your life.
- It is perennial wisdom that the capacity to think is a great servant but a terrible master when you exercise no control over it.

# Chapter 10

## *Pleasure anxiety*

## Catastrophic thinking and *pleasure anxiety* are kissing cousins

*Pleasure anxiety* refers to a conditioned aversion toward pleasure because pleasure triggers a fear that something bad might happen if one is feeling good and unprepared for danger. *Pleasure anxiety* shows up in the core thought, "If I feel good, I am not safe."

Pleasure anxiety can reach the level of terror in some individuals and the relaxation protocol must be modified to help someone through this anxiety. How I have seen this work in *Paradoxical Relaxation* is that sometimes, as people with pleasure anxiety follow the relaxation instructions and the nervous system begins to quiet down, their hearts begin to beat faster, their palms begin to sweat and, to their distress, they feel more anxious as their nervous system begins to quiet down during the relaxation session. This reaction is a heightened psycho physical defense against letting down their guard and vigilance and feeling good. The warning signal goes off saying that danger is occurring because something is feeling good and vigilance is being relaxed.

Pleasure anxiety shows up in the core thought, "If I feel good, I am not safe"

People with a chronically *upregulated nervous system* tends to seek something to worry about to justify their arousal when one worry has been resolved. If you are chronically anxious, friends or family may notice that you are always worried about something. Once one worry goes away, you quickly find another to replace it. If you have pleasure anxiety, when you reflect upon your life, you may notice that it is very rare for you to feel good for more than a few hours or a day. This may or may not be immediately obvious to you because you are so used to going from worry to worry in the drama of your life, though others close to you may often notice and are puzzled by it.

## Identifying the thought, "If I feel good, I am not safe"

Anxiety and anxiety-related disorders tend to be part of the habit of conditioned vigilance. This vigilance says, "Beyond a certain point, it is not safe for me to relax, feel good, safe, happy, free, unguarded." Chronic anxiety is often the expression of an early conditioning that says, "If I am not on my guard, I am in danger."

Almost universally, chronically anxious individuals bump up against a stubborn barrier to quieting down, to relaxing their muscle tension and allowing their level of arousal and guardedness to release. This stubborn barrier to relaxation is not arbitrary. This kind of thought is typically conditioned early in life and it is why relaxation beyond a certain point can be scary. I discuss this later in describing the formation of the inner *tyrannical caretaker*, which attempts to forbid any possibility of vulnerability to the kind of past trauma or pain that has occurred.

Here is an example of pleasure anxiety. A patient with pelvic pain experienced the death of her mother at a time in her life when the patient was happy and carefree. The news of her mother's death occurred suddenly and shocked her. From the time of her mother's death she remained nervous and wary. Although she was rarely consciously aware of this, deep in her mind, the experience of being happy and carefree was somehow connected to a terrible event happening.

It was for this reason she complained that she could never relax. She reported to her psychotherapist that as she grew older and explored her life, she seemed to be uncomfortable feeling good. She reported that invariably when she felt a sense of contentment, negative thoughts about bad things that might happen in the future would come to her mind and her good mood evaporated. Moreover, she reported that she felt strangely naked when her pelvic pain would subside. Her treatment involved a focus on tolerating pleasure and accepting the absence of anxiety. This was no small enterprise.

## Relaxing with pleasure anxiety

While this kind of reaction often prompts the person experiencing it to stop doing relaxation, on the contrary, perseverance through this reaction is vital. However, instead of fighting the defense, one must be gentle with it.

There is a parable that is instructive.

> *The north wind and the sun were arguing about who was more powerful. During their argument they both spotted a man who was wearing a winter coat. The north wind proposed a wager with the sun as to who could better get the man to take the coat off. "You go first," said the sun and so the north wind blew hard and cold on the man with a warm fur jacket. The harder the north wind blew, the more desperately the man put his arms around himself, holding more tightly to his jacket. Exhausted, the north wind looked at the sun with frustration and said, "There is no way anyone can part this man from his jacket." The sun just smiled and said, "We'll see." Then the sun shone on the man, radiating more and more warmth in his direction. The man with the coat relaxed and let go of his desperate clutching. As the sun continued to shine, the man unbuttoned his coat. Finally, turning toward the sun's warmth, the man took off his jacket.*

Force typically hardens fear-based resistance. The stubborn clutching based on the fear of not being on guard does not loosen with force. As the north wind discovered, force tends to harden clutching. As the man in the parable responded to the warmth of the sun by taking off the protection of his coat, so the conditioned inner defenses that fear being undefended, respond to an inner attitude of kindness, gentleness, and compassion. In other words, your own *compassionate* regard for your fear of feeling safe can loosen this fear.

By remaining still and *even considering* focusing attention away from worry and guardedness when doing *Paradoxical Relaxation*, some patients feel that they are jumping out of their skin. In dealing with extreme pleasure anxiety and the idea that it is not safe to be undefended, it is sometimes necessary to reduce the duration of the relaxation session to a period of one or two minutes so that the subconscious resistance can discover that it is safe to quiet down even for this very short period. As one can tolerate more time of reduced arousal, one increases the duration of the relaxation session. It is a delicate dance and it is important for the person dealing with pleasure anxiety who does *Paradoxical Relaxation* to rely on someone who understands what is going on and can be a guide through it.

## The *great impasse-opportunity*: resting with the fear response in you that says it isn't safe to let go

It is a remarkable moment when you are face to face with a pattern of tension that has been going on unconsciously most of your life. I want to call that moment the *great impasse-opportunity.* It is the moment during a relaxation session when you are resting with the tension in you, discussed in chapter 6 as the *default inner posture,* that has been there for a very long time and that you have not been able to release.

In the moment, while resting with the *great impasse-opportunity*, you must be willing to never feel better. In the moment of the relaxation session, it is very helpful to assume the attitude of being willing to simply rest in the impasse forever. This is a trick to defeat this impasse but paradoxically there can be no intention to defeat the impasse when you practice adopting the willingness for the impasse to never go away.

It is a peculiar inner strategy and, in my experience, the only one I have found that has allowed this impasse to dissolve. Allowing the resistance in you to remain and taking the attitude that it is okay that it remains forever is what can dissolve the impasse. Again, this is a profound paradox.

## Practicing *Paradoxical Relaxation* means practicing not worrying: the tale of tasting the strawberry

The following parable tells the story of letting go of worry in the most extreme of moments. It is a story about the fearlessness of living life in the midst of impossible obstacles. In the moment of doing *Paradoxical Relaxation*, it is the practice of not knowing what is going to happen in your life and relaxing anyway.

> *A man was chased to the edge of a cliff by two hungry tigers. Just as the tigers were about to pounce on him, he saw a vine growing at the edge of the cliff, grabbed it and moved down far enough on the vine to escape the jaws of the tigers. The man looked down to the bottom of the cliff and saw a hundred hungry tigers looking up at him waiting for him to fall so that they could have their mid-day lunch. Above, the man saw two mice gnawing away at the vine onto which he was holding.*
>
> *When the man looked at the face of the cliff, within his reach he saw a wild strawberry growing. He looked at the tigers below and the gnawing mice above, then shrugged his shoulders, reached out to the face of the cliff and plucked the wild strawberry. He popped the strawberry in his mouth. Tasting it with delight, he said, "How sweet."*

In the practice of *Paradoxical Relaxation* we are often letting go of guarding in the middle of unresolved circumstances where we are caught between mice gnawing at the vine holding us above and hungry tigers below.

## Using *Paradoxical Relaxation* in moments of uncertainty and anxiety

When I feel like the man hanging from the vine off of a cliff, I practice *Paradoxical Relaxation*. Doing *Paradoxical Relaxation* at such a time requires that I take my attention away from my worrisome and catastrophic thoughts, away from the hungry tigers, the gnawing mice and the uncertainty of how my life feels in that moment, in order to bring myself back into peace.

Taking my attention away from my worrisome thoughts is a profound existential decision

Taking attention away from worrisome or catastrophic thinking during *Paradoxical Relaxation* is the practice of ceasing to pay attention to your scary thinking in the presence of uncertainty. *Practicing Paradoxical Relaxation during periods of worry or fears of catastrophe is the practice of choosing not to worry.*

When I work with a patient who compulsively catastrophizes and worries, I recognize that patient in me. This is the part of me that says, under the circumstances of what is going on and the future isn't clear, it is not safe to stop worrying, even for a moment. This part of me says it is necessary to keep vigilant and fearful. Under these circumstances, it isn't safe to feel safe.

When I find myself compulsively worrying or catastrophizing like this, the worrier in me doesn't want me to stop focusing on what is scary. While I don't exactly talk to myself this way, if I were to give words to my decision to stop worrying, this is what would I say to the part of me glued to worrisome thoughts:

> *"I understand you hate uncertainty and you are imagining bad things happening. I understand that you think that keeping me worrying without a break is your way of protecting me.*
>
> *I have done everything I can do to rationally evaluate whether your worrisome and catastrophic thinking is true, and have gone as far as I can go in reassuring you. I understand that you think that it is not safe for me to stop worrying, even for a moment.*

*Your worry has motivated me to take certain constructive action and I appreciate you for motivating me to do this. I have taken every possible action to take care of the situation. I always do. I have made the phone calls, written what needed to be written, called whomever should be called, put in place every precaution that should be taken. And in the next 45 minutes, there is no value in my continuing to be in fear.*

*Your compulsion to have me focus my attention on thoughts that are worrisome every moment, and particularly in the next 45 minutes makes no sense to me, and it will keep me tired and miserable. And I see that calming down and bringing myself back into peace during this relaxation session makes the most sense. Continually worrying in the next 45 minutes offers me nothing except suffering.*

*For these reasons, I am choosing to give myself a break in the next 45 minutes. I am going to rest my attention in sensation and stop focusing on what is worrisome. This means that I am choosing to stop worrying. I know you may not be comfortable with this. I am going to rest with your discomfort about me stopping worrying as well."*

I have found great value in an abbreviated form of this kind of inner dialogue that precedes a relaxation session in the middle of anxiety and uncertainty.

## Recognizing the resistance to being hopeful again when a catastrophic thought goes away

You would think that the anxious patient would want to feel relief after a catastrophic thought goes away. It is not uncommon, however, for anxious patients to be reluctant to allow themselves to feel relief when a catastrophic thought resolves or a situation that they were catastrophizing about goes away. When I have explored this phenomenon with some anxious patients, the catastrophizing part of the personality doesn't want to give up its vigilance.

## Putting a period at the end of an episode of worry

Some people don't want to feel good again once the catastrophic thought has passed and has been proven wrong. This is usually because the old defense against disappointment reasserts itself and doesn't want to be surprised by something bad happening for which it is not prepared. The irrational logic of this idea is that it is better to be anxious and vigilant all of the time than to stop being vigilant and get caught off guard by a new, potentially catastrophic event. This idea is absurd because, carried to its logical conclusion, all it will do is keep you miserable your whole life so that you are not surprised by misery.

If you do not let go of the vigilant state once the worried thought has been resolved, you rob yourself of the opportunity to truly rest and be worry free. In the absence of something to worry about, there is no reason for the vigilant, fearful state.

## Increased periods of peace of mind are the best medicine for chronic anxiety

In the strategy of dissolving the grip of the core thought that it isn't safe to feel safe, it can be helpful to increase the number of *Paradoxical Relaxation* sessions. If the problem of chronic anxiety is a hyper-aroused (upregulated) nervous system, the 'medicine' is increasing the duration you are able to voluntarily calm down your nervous system. This is most easily and deliberately achieved by doing sessions of *Paradoxical Relaxation*. During that time you can devote yourself to taking attention away from disturbing thinking and resting attention in sensation.

## ***Paradoxical Relaxation*** is the practice of choosing to allow the feeling of openness and vulnerability

*The practice of Paradoxical Relaxation is the practice of allowing yourself to be at ease, to feel good, and to let go of vigilance.* Sometimes patients experience feeling good and release from vigilance as a feeling of openness and vulnerability. Our treatment bumps up against psychological patterns that refuse to let go of psychological defenses. When patients are at a plateau in which their symptoms stop improving it is often helpful to facilitate a dialogue, commonly used in Gestalt therapy, between the part of the patient that wants to improve and the part that seems unable to move ahead. What often emerges from these dialogues is the fear of the unknown, the fear of being open and vulnerable.

## When you've been in a dark room for a long time, it can be scary to come out into the light

> *When I was in college I had a cat named Licker, so named by the neighborhood children because he was fond of licking everything in sight. One day I had to take Licker to the vet for his shots and I constructed a cat-box in order to transport him in my car. He fought and scratched me with remarkable energy as he resisted me putting him in the cat-box. He remained in the cat-box for about 8 hours and I suffered along with him in his distress over being confined. When I got home with him after the visit to the vet, I eagerly opened the door to the cat-box, grateful to be able to free him from his prison. To my surprise, he did not rush out as I had expected him to. Instead he remained in the cat-box, huddled in the corner.*
>
> *It took my cat some time to leave the cat-box. He was wary as he approached the door. It was as if the environment where he was free and able to easily move about in had become foreign to him. After he left the cat-box and resumed his life as an unconfined cat, he reverted back to his normal*

> *behavior. Strangely, it seems, he had gotten used to being in that little cat prison.*

For those whose habit is to compulsively worry, the idea that feeling safe is not safe and can be scary, is like the cat-box was for my cat. *Staying in the cat-box is a compulsive focus on worrisome thoughts.* My cat's coming back into the freedom of being out of the cage can be compared to relearning that it is okay to not worry in this moment. *Coming out of the cat-box is the willingness to risk that feeling safe is safe.*

Often I will ask someone who has this tendency, to feel that part of them that is reiterating the worrisome thought over and over again. I will say, "Feel the part of you that is telling the other part of you what is worrisome." Most people are able to feel that part of the themselves. As the part of them that I might call 'the worrier' communicates the worry, I will say, "Turn your attention to this part of you. I want to ask the worrier in you some questions." "What if the other part of you released its vigilance right now?" The worrier part of the person will typically then say, "Something bad would happen. We wouldn't be prepared for the danger. It isn't safe to stop worrying." When I have asked the worrier part of the person, "Is it ever safe to feel safe?" the worrier usually says, "No."

The repetitive use of *Paradoxical Relaxation* can begin to break the grip of this compulsive worrying. The instruction is to take attention away from any worrisome thought, over and over again. In the moment of being caught in compulsive worry, by using *Paradoxical Relaxation*, the person who is afraid to feel safe can sometimes break the compulsive focus on what is scary.

## Worry has to do with focusing attention on what is worrisome

Worry is a certain kind of focus of attention. When you worry, your attention is focused on thoughts that scare you. When you take your attention off of such thoughts...in that moment you stop worrying. Simple. Most of the time, when you think catastrophically and you go around in a state of continual worry, this worry is dysfunctional. It serves no purpose. It doesn't help you protect yourself or take care of your life. It tends to just keep you scared and miserable. So the practice of taking attention away from worry is a practice of disidentifying with the part of you who has chosen to believe that it is not safe to feel safe.

> When individuals are prone to worry, the core thought they have had for a long time tends to be that they are safest when they worry

When you do *Paradoxical Relaxation*, you are practicing focusing your attention on sensation and away from thought. The central instruction of *Paradoxical Relaxation* is that when you find your attention focusing on a thought—any thought—your job is to take your attention off of the thought over and over again. *The most important point here is that when you practice Paradoxical Relaxation, you practice controlling your attention so that it is not paying attention to thought of any kind.*

When you direct your attention away from a thought, you are exercising an act of will that says to the part of you insisting on focusing on worrisome thoughts, "At this time, I do not want to listen to you. I do not want to pay attention to you. I don't want to enter into the world that you portray. At this moment I don't want to heed you. With no malice I turn away from you. I choose not to think, which means I don't want to focus on my thoughts."

When you first begin the practice of *Paradoxical Relaxation*, attention is usually very difficult to control and there is usually a compulsive and involuntary focus of attention on thinking of all kinds, from trivial to catastrophic.

## Trusting that it is okay to take your attention off of what is worrisome

Practicing taking attention away from the worrisome or catastrophic thinking represents a conscious choice, a conscious refusal to believe one of the premises of your conditioning which is that you are only safe if you focus on what is worrisome or catastrophic because if you don't, you are setting yourself up to be surprised and unprepared for the bad that can happen.

Taking this existential position is a major moment in life. It is taking the risk of not letting your conditioning control you. It is a moment of trusting that it is safe for you to allow yourself and the world to be as they are, and in that moment you don't have to do anything about what is… you can just let it be.

This moment often happens after someone has experienced a catastrophic event like a heart attack, a terminal diagnosis, or a near death experience, and they feel released of the need to worry anymore. The worst has happened and here you are. I have had more than one friend say that having cancer was the best thing that ever happened to them. How unfortunate that we often have to have such events occur to release ourselves from our irrational concept of what it takes to remain safe.

I am not suggesting that if there is a fire in your house and the thoughts that arise in your mind having to do with putting out the fire and protecting yourself from it be ignored. On the contrary, it is essential to use your mind skillfully to deal with emergencies and difficulties in life. Most compulsive worriers are very skillful and competent in dealing with difficulties in life that arise.

Disidentification from the worrier part of your personality means that you see yourself as more than this small part of your personality. For example, when you compulsively worry, the part of you who is the worrier, who believes that it is not safe to feel safe, usually has sway over your life and your attention. When you disidentify from this part, you tell yourself that this response in you is not the essential you. You tell yourself that it is a part of you that is conditioned by past circumstances and is deluded and unreliable in this moment. This disidentification can help free you from the continual obligation of the worrier in you to focus attention on what is worrisome.

## Disidentification from the worrier is like the practice of walking out of a bad movie or choosing not to eat a bad meal

Disidentification from the worrier in you is not something that just happens. *Disidentification from the worrier must be repeatedly practiced. You get better at it as you practice it.* And the skill of disidentification takes years to develop. It must be practiced, often poorly, over and over again until you get good at it. As you take your attention off of one catastrophic or negative thought after the other, over and over and over again, it is like the practice of walking out of a bad movie and not feeling compelled to stay through the whole thing just because you paid for it.

As you practice walking out of bad movies, you get better at it. You recognize the bad movie very soon into it and you more and more easily get out of your seat and leave the theatre. When you practice disidentification with the worrier, you get better at identifying the catastrophic thinking sooner and letting it go sooner. But it takes a long time and requires patience and faith.

When you practice disidentification from the worrier, you are saying to the worrier, "Beyond doing everything I need to be doing about what is worrisome, I no longer have use for you. I no longer want to follow what makes you comfortable which is always insisting that I keep my attention on what is worrisome."

### The thinking mind isn't ashamed to think anything

When I see people first begin on the great journey of taking control of their thoughts, some become angry or judgmental with themselves for thinking the way they do. Years ago when I first began to explore my own thinking and was honest with myself, I routinely found irrational and stubborn thinking coexisted with my rational, wise, and carefully considered way of thinking. As I have spent many years looking into my thinking and how it is the major source of my suffering in life, I have been able to find some compassion for myself. I have found irony and compassion in Byron Katie's observation that the mind isn't ashamed to think anything.

Here is a typical example from my own life. A friend was brusque with me and the thought arose in my mind that she was angry with me or didn't like me anymore. My story to myself about my friend's reaction made me the center of my friend's reaction. Inevitably, I spoke to my friend, shared my feelings and thoughts about her brusqueness and discovered that my friend was having a hard time about something that had nothing to do with me. My friend told me that she was enduringly devoted to me and loved me. I saw that I made up the whole story about her in my mind, and I smiled ironically to myself. For the ten-thousandth time I saw how my mind wasn't ashamed to think anything.

When I see my mind operating this way, which it often does, these days I am amused. I am not shocked. I am not judgmental. *I don't take my irrational thinking personally.*

I have come to see that to let go of irrational thinking, it is helpful to not take your irrational thinking personally. If you negatively judge yourself for your irrational thinking, you will have a harder time in letting go of this thinking.

I have learned to have compassion for myself in having thoughts that scare me or make me miserable. I have become much more able to make the distinction between reality and catastrophic thoughts when they first occur.

To know that you are a prisoner of your own mind and live in an imaginary world of your own creation is the dawn of wisdom

Nisargadatta said that it is a mark of maturity to become aware of how we confuse our thinking for reality. He was saying that a less developed stage of personal and spiritual development is when you don't know the difference between your irrational and catastrophic thinking and reality.

Recognizing that your unexamined and unmanaged thinking is the source of your imprisonment is a very positive sign, a sign that you are on the right road. It is the dawn of wisdom. If you don't see the source of your suffering as your tendency to catastrophize and make up stories that make you miserable, you continue to suffer.

## Not taking your fear of feeling safe personally

There are things that other people have to deal with that you don't, but the tendency toward anxiety and the fear of feeling safe may be what you have to deal with. It is most helpful to not take this tendency personally as it is just something that comes with the package that is you. Judging yourself about this tendency is purely optional and discretionary. If you want to stop doing it, you can.

Consider thinking that working with this issue of getting hijacked by irrational thoughts is a part of your curriculum in life. It is not something that can just get immediately cured. You live with it and work with it in order to find your way out of it. As you work with your thinking, you'll find out what works and what doesn't and you'll notice the life cycle of your catastrophic thinking. Fearful thinking that paints the world as a place in which you can never feel safe has a beginning, middle, and end. I think it is most helpful to set the goal of making the distance between the beginning and the end of fearful thinking shorter and shorter.

Freeing yourself from fear is the most important thing you can do to live a happy life

Extricating ourselves from the fear of feeling safe and undefended is not unlike my cat's journey of getting used to being free again after its confinement in the cat box in which I had carried it to the vet. The first step is to recognize the attachment one part of us has to staying afraid in order to feel safe.

I often tell people who struggle with the core belief that "it isn't safe to feel safe" that they don't have to take this belief personally. Most people are perplexed by this comment. What I mean by not taking it personally is this: people who suffer from anxiety typically have a *certain conditioning* and perhaps even some genetic inclination that predisposes them in one degree or another toward anxiety and the fear of being without fear. Given a different mother and father and childhood or different genes, the issue of anxiety may not have ever shown up. Our essential nature is peaceful even if we have a predisposition to anxiety. *Whatever it's source, anxiety interferes with the experience of our natural state.*

In a sense this predisposition is like having blue eyes or brown hair. It is a tendency you didn't choose, and would choose differently if you could. The tendency doesn't mean that you must be driven or controlled by it. It simply means that it is there and has to be attended to and tamed. It is just part of the hand you were dealt and you have the opportunity to not be imprisoned by such a tendency.

## Forgiving the part of you that holds irrational beliefs

Not taking the fear of feeling safe personally is particularly important for people who judge themselves negatively for what they view to be irrational thinking. Negative self-judgment is entirely unhelpful and actually interferes with your ability to better deal with catastrophic, it-is not-safe-to-feel-safe thinking. I tell people to consider being interested in, and not judgmental of their tendency to catastrophize.

## The great existential question: is it safe in this moment to feel safe?

When is it safe to feel safe? When is it okay to feel that everything is okay? Is it safe to not be anxious if I genuinely don't know what is going to happen in my life tomorrow, if the world is crazy and unpredictable? Is it safe to feel safe in the middle of feelings of anxiety if I am in pain? And even if it is safe to feel safe right now, for how long is it safe to feel safe?

Is it okay in this moment not to be anxious when the world is a crazy place with so many things going on that could be catastrophic?

These questions are uncommon. These questions, however, as strange as they sound on the surface, are ongoing unresolved questions of many anxious people who struggle with pleasure anxiety or catastrophic thinking. They are not to be questions of the rational intellect. There is a deep confusion and uncertainty— often unspoken—in most people who suffer from anxiety as to when it is okay to feel safe.

In every relaxation session, you come face to face with the question of when is it safe to feel safe. In each relaxation session, you have the opportunity to answer 'now' to this question

*Paradoxical Relaxation* asks you to let go of any circumstances or rationalizations that say it is not safe to be safe now. In *Paradoxical Relaxation*, you are asked to be okay now, with what is, including the part of you that is tight and defends against what is.

The *Serenity Prayer* in Alcoholics Anonymous is a prayer answering this question. It says:

Give me the ability to change what I can change,
The knowledge to accept what I can't change,
And the wisdom to know the difference

The truth is that the only person who can ultimately give you permission to be okay with what is going on now, is you. Every authority, every wise person, can say it is or is not okay to feel okay with *what is* but ultimately you get to decide how you want to be around *what is.* This is a question around which you ultimately have the final freedom of choice.

The truth is that you are the only person who can ultimately give yourself permission to be okay with what is going on now. In Paradoxical Relaxation, you get to choose whether you put the Serenity Prayer into action. In a session of Paradoxical Relaxation, you have the question put to you every moment as to whether it is okay to change what you can control and accept what you can't control and be at peace with it all

In my own life, it is my intention to be okay with that over which I have no control. And if I can't seem to get myself to be okay with something that is, it is my intention to be okay with my inability to get myself to be okay.

When is it okay not to be anxious? My answer is: always

I heard a story about someone who was at a dinner party during the war in Lebanon at the height of a very violent period. Gunfire could be heard in the distance. The hostess came into her living room and said to her guests quite plainly, "Well, we can wait until the war is over, or we can have dinner." This somehow puts it very well.

When is it okay not to be anxious? My answer is: always.

# Chapter 11

## *Dissolving inner resistance to relaxation by accepting the inner resistance*

Relaxation is easy and needs no special training. Dealing with resistance to relaxation is what Paradoxical Relaxation training is all about

It is easy to relax a tightened fist you have just made. You tighten the muscles and now they relax easily when you decide to let go of tightening them. What is not obvious and outside the ability of most people is to voluntarily relax contracted muscles and an aroused nervous system that is not cooperating with your wish to relax them. "Resistance" is the name you can give to the refusal of your body at any particular level to relax. This refusal is usually quite primitive and on the level of a two year old saying "no." It is generally not a good idea in parenting to use unkind force to make a two year old bend to your will. Similarly, you cannot unkindly force an aroused nervous system to relax.

The only way I have been able to defeat inner resistance to letting go is to accept it

The resistance to letting go defends against relaxation. I am clear that there is no way to cheat this defense. In my view, it is unlikely that hypnotizing someone and waving the magic wand of therapeutic suggestion, for example, or giving medication, doing surgery, or using other interventions that work from the outside to the inside, will bypass or short-circuit this conditioned resistance.

## Resistance in relaxation has similarities to the resistances found in people suffering from trauma

Most of us forget how emotionally open and vulnerable we were as children. We forget how deeply life affected us on a moment to moment basis. We forget, as very young children, our intense grief at the thought of being abandoned when our parents left the room and were out of our sight. We forget that we didn't understand the idea of the future, because as children we were forever living in the present moment. In that eternal present, we forget how it felt when our parents left us at home with a caregiver, not understanding that they would return. We forget the bone-chilling terror and sense of devastation of a mother or a father's angry displeasure with us. When we hear the heart wrenching cry of an infant that pulls on us to go toward it to console it, we forget that the infant once was us.

As adults we tend to forget the state we were in as young children when we had no barrier and no shield against the immediate and intimate tornado of our own emotions or those of others. When those emotions were loving and positive, we could experience the joy, peace and bliss described in fairy tales. When those emotions were negative or threatening, we could experience a terror that made us feel like we were on the verge of annihilation.

The remembrance of this childhood universe can help clarify the stubbornness of the resistances to relaxation many experience in practicing *Paradoxical Relaxation.* Donald Kalsched's exploration of early childhood trauma is instructive. When the infant or young child is faced with what we now call abuse or trauma, as Kalsched movingly discusses in his book, *The Inner World of Trauma*, a primitive, self-protective reaction occurs to protect the overwhelmed child. Kalsched variously names this reaction a *protector/persecutor*, or a *tyrannical caretaker.* He suggests that this reaction that occurs within a young, traumatized child is indeed the reaction of a *tyrannical caretaker*, whose mission is self-protective but eventually misguided and self destructive. He writes:

> *"This primitive (tyrannical, caretaking) defense does not learn anything about realistic danger as the child grows up. It functions on the magical level of consciousness with the same level of awareness it had when the original trauma or traumas occurred. Each new life opportunity (to open, grow, and love) is mistakenly seen as a dangerous threat of retraumatization and is therefore attacked...."*

Kalsched goes on to describe the ferocity of this inner protective reaction in its single-minded intention to protect whatever vestige of trust in life survived the overwhelming trauma. He describes this peculiar and yet self-destructive tendency of the psyche to prevent *even the possibility* of further trauma by banishing any inner vulnerability to being surprised by the kind of pain that was once experienced.

In other words, when someone was deeply hurt as a very young child, a peculiar and ostensibly self protective reaction sometimes can enduringly remain to protect from the surprise of being hurt again. This reaction explains the behavior of certain people who seem to sabotage every relationship that they are ever in because this reaction can't permit them to become vulnerable to the possibility of being hurt. This primitive reaction says that it is better to remain closed to dependency and intimacy than risk being open, vulnerable, dependent, and suffer from what assault might occur when in such an unprotected and vulnerable state. Kalsched writes:

> *"Never again" says our tyrannical caretaker, "will the traumatized personal spirit of (my inner) child suffer this badly! Never again will (I) be this helpless in the face of cruel reality...before this happens I will disperse into fragments (dissociation) or encapsulate it and soothe it with fantasy (schizoid withdrawal) or numb it with intoxicating substances (addiction) or persecute it to keep it from hoping for life in this world (depression)...in this way I will preserve what is left of this permanently amputated childhood—of an innocence that has suffered too much too soon."*

When the inner experience of a very young child is too painful for the young child to process, a self protective reaction forms as a defense. Any inner experience of vulnerability or openness feels like the vulnerability and openness in childhood when the traumas and pain occurred. "If I forbid myself to be vulnerable, unguarded and unafraid, I am safe." I characterized this psychic inner strategy when I described pleasure anxiety.

Kalsched characterizes the different ways that a human being defends against the feeling of vulnerability and openness after an unresolved trauma by using categories of dissociation, schizoid withdrawal, addiction and depression. In fact, the defense against vulnerability after trauma is not confined to these categories. The tendency to obsess and keep attention focused on a single idea is also a way of defending against the scary vulnerability of something bad happening again. What is called an *ear worm* or tune that goes around and around in your head, can also be considered obsessive thinking and may perform the same function of defending against the feeling of vulnerability,

What Kalsched calls the *tyrannical caretaker* can be labeled a subpersonality, a defensive reaction, a splinter from the psyche, an enduring characterological post-traumatic stress disorder, or simply a defensive resistance to deep relaxation. As I discuss below, the resistance to fully relaxing, which Jacobson called the residual tension, when given words, turns out to be the *tyrannical caretaker.* The *tyrannical caretaker* happens to be expressed physically in what I describe as the *default inner posture* as well as psychologically in what I describe as *pleasure anxiety.*

Again, the defensive resistance to relaxation, whether it is called the *default inner posture, pleasure anxiety,* the *tyrannical caretaker,* a psychic splinter or subpersonality, or a characterological post-traumatic stress disorder, all sing the same tune. These terms are all descriptions, from different vantage points, of the same inner phenomenon. The script reads, "If I feel safe, unafraid, spontaneous, unguarded, I am not safe but in danger. I will not allow myself to be exposed and vulnerable to being surprised at being hurt. I might be hurt or rejected but I will not be surprised by it."

The tyrannical caretaker defense does not just exist in people who have been traumatized... individuals who never experience trauma, who simply deal with the garden-variety suffering of childhood can develop this same fierce kind of inner defense. The tyrannical caretaker shows up physically in the form of the default inner posture

You don't have to be horribly abused to feel, "It is not safe for me to feel safe" or, "I cannot allow myself to completely relax." This inner script, in fact, occurs in people who have not been abused, as well as in those who have. *The inner experience of defending against deep relaxation in the non-abused person can be just as fierce as in the abused person.*

## The strategy of *Paradoxical Relaxation* is to bring into awareness, and become friends again with the part of ourselves that refuses to relax

The lie of the *tyrannical caretaker* is that remaining closed off, vigilant, and anxious will protect you from bad things happening. At best, the *tyrannical caretaker* kind of vigilance will mitigate the surprise at bad things happening. It can't stop bad things from happening. If I remain vigilant, anxious and tensed, I behave like I am in a fight and am defending myself against a blow that I am not able to escape. Can I stop the blow by tightening up? No. I can stop it from hurting me as much as if I were relaxed and not defended against it.

The *tyrannical caretaker* defense does not want to hear that it cannot stop the blow. It is not interested in the facts. It is a kind of hysterical, unreasoning clamping down, to gain some control over fates that can't be controlled. It trades joy, spontaneity, softness, love, openness and peace for a bogus sense of security in which it demands that we remain eternally afraid. It promotes the idea that you can be safe by always being reminded that you are never safe. It indeed is a blind and unreasoning attempt to gain some sense of control of life by promoting us to remain fearful of what might happen. It attempts to guard against what it ultimately can't stop by demanding we live a miserable and joyless life of worry.

The *tyrannical caretaker* defense sees relaxation as dangerous, as a state in which you have no control over bad things. And yet no matter how hard it forces you to tighten up, or how long it stops you from letting go, it ultimately has no control over the whims of fate. If anything, in causing you to be chronically tensed and anxious, the *tyrannical caretaker* defense promotes less competent judgment and ability to act. It distracts your attention from what you are doing, it keeps your nervous system in a fight-flight-freeze mode eventually compromising your immune system, it makes you less attractive as a human being to others because of your joylessness and anxiety, and most important it robs you of your inner peace. Most people never examine or challenge their inner *tyrannical caretaker.*

Most people who do *Paradoxical Relaxation* do not feel connected to the fact that they are the agent of the defensive tension in them that refuses to relax. The *tyrannical caretaker* defense is typically unconscious. When people get in touch with it and learn about it, they are very often stunned by it. When this tension is given words, as I ask patients to give their residual tension words when I help them identify their *default inner posture*, the purpose of this tension makes no sense.

The *tyrannical caretaker* defense is usually harsh, unyielding, ruthless, and irrational. When you confront this part of the personality with the fact that ultimately the tension that is forced on the body cannot stop bad things happening, it turns a deaf ear. It is not interested. "Don't confuse me with the facts" appears to be its viewpoint. If bad things happen, it wants us to be prepared. It is a primitive defensive reaction. It is unmoved by what by any standard is reasonable, loving and good. It has far more affinity to the style of Sadaam Hussein than to the style of Mahatma Gandhi.

When asked if there is ever a moment when it is okay to completely let go and be unguarded, the inner resistance will typically say "Never." Having fun is not in its vocabulary. Hanging out is not in its vocabulary. It is all business—in the service of survival, of protecting the person by being on guard and not surprised by pain or danger. It refuses to accept the inherent transiency and uncertainty in life. For this defensive reaction, the end of not being surprised by bad things justifies the means of being brutal, inflicting pain, fear and suffering on oneself if that is what it takes to not be surprised.

Fritz Perls, in Gestalt therapy, routinely worked with these kinds of defensive reactions with the understanding that 'them is us.' In Gestalt therapy, these unconscious responses and attitudes that defeat us in our life need to be made conscious and 're-owned.' The re-owning of the *tyrannical caretaker* means that we take it back as part of us. It no longer is a *thing*, separate inside of us, that cannot be released.

Indeed, the *tyrannical caretaker* is not a thing, not a demon inhabiting us. *It is simply a deep dysfunctional and primitive reaction that we must not go to war against if we want to become free of it.* If we go to war against the *tyrannical caretaker* or any other unconscious and primitive reaction inside, we harden it. Like the story of the north wind and the sun betting who could get the man to take off his coat, we want to get this reaction of refusal to let go in us, to 'take its coat off' by the warmth of the sun and not the harsh force of the north wind. We want to reabsorb the energy of the *tyrannical caretaker* back into ourselves where it is no longer separate and dark.

## The psychological strategy behind *Paradoxical Relaxation* is the practice of loving kindness toward oneself

*When you look at the resistance to relaxation in this way—as a self protective reaction aimed at protecting oneself from being unguarded in the face of something bad happening, the strategy of Paradoxical Relaxation becomes clear.* Facing the dilemma of what to do with the tyrannical caretaker is what many people who wish to learn *Paradoxical Relaxation* have to face. *The strategy of Paradoxical Relaxation is a strategy of loving kindness to this old terrified reaction in oneself. In my view is the only effective way to deal with this distressing and debilitating primitive reaction.*

In *Paradoxical Relaxation*, we practice behaving toward our resistance as the kindest, most loving and patient parent we can possibly imagine. We bring continuous, unconditional attention to the part of us that is fearful, guarded, and unamenable to reason. We practice loving kindness to a part of us that screams *no* to life, love, openness, joy and freedom. We make no demands on this part of us. We do not force or cajole or try to push this part of us beyond what it is comfortable within the moment. And we don't allow our attention to be held captive by the *tyrannical caretaker.* In *Paradoxical Relaxation*, we assert our will by resting our attention in sensation despite the protests of this inner part of us that doesn't want attention to be taken away from worrisome, vigilant thoughts.

It is with the strategy of profound, focused and devoted attention, giving up all attachment to an outcome, that this terrified and resistant part of us can lay down its hopeless mission and allow us to open up our hearts, to let go of defending against our experience of being. In various forms, this has been the strategy of the deepest practices of the wisdom traditions throughout the ages.

## Not fighting with the rebel in you

A battle against the *tyrannical caretaker* in you will stalemate your relaxation practice. Such confrontation consumes energy and keeps the nervous system aroused. The key to ending this battle with the part of you that doesn't want to cooperate with the relaxation instructions is to notice and immediately accept it. What this has meant in practical terms in my own practice is that when I feel resistance to the subtle activity of accepting the discomfort, I simply feel this tightening. Most importantly I make it okay that nothing has to happen. I continue the practice with the idea that it is fine if I never relax.

In other words, in allowing the resistance to accepting the tension, you may become aware of feeling the unpleasant sensations of restlessness or impatience. When you hear the instruction that says that it is okay to feel unpleasant sensations, in wanting to do the method correctly, you notice any part of you that does not want to play this game. The rebellious part of you that is wordless when it comes into your awareness, if it had words to speak would say, "I don't want to feel that." This resistance to feeling the unpleasant sensation usually shows up as a certain kind of tension in you.

## Accepting both the anxiety and discomfort in your body and the rebel in you who does not want to feel the anxiety and discomfort

Here is the point. During relaxation, while resting attention in sensation you want to accept everything—both the anxiety and discomfort in your body and the part of you that does not want to feel the discomfort. You must learn to allow both to be present. This acceptance doesn't mean you are going to love anxiety and resistance. It simply means that you allow the presence of what does not feel particularly good as well as allowing your dislike of what doesn't feel particularly good. This is a dynamic process that will change moment by moment. You permit all the resistances to arise that fight against the intention that you are setting to focus your attention. You permit whatever arises, including the resistance to permitting what arises.

Permitting aversion and resistance to what you are adverse to goes against the general orientation in our culture regarding what to do with pain. This instruction says your job during relaxation is *not* to take an aspirin, not to distract yourself, not to eat, smoke, drink, have sex, or do anything to get away from the discomfort that you are feeling. Instead, the instruction is to turn toward the discomfort without attachment or aversion. The instruction is to rest *alongside* of the tension or discomfort. On a moment by moment basis, the idea is to renounce trying to get anywhere or trying to make the discomfort better.

## Getting comfortable with what isn't comfortable

The only amelioration of discomfort you might seek during the relaxation session is to get more comfortable and relaxed with what is uncomfortable and what is not relaxed. This type of instruction is often difficult to understand and put into practice by the novice. Yet, it is the key to profound states of relaxation.

This must be practiced over and over again as it is the only real way to follow this instruction. Again, the acceptance of what is uncomfortable is most likely to transform the discomfort into what is comfortable. The paradox is that you generally have to give up your attachment to feeling comfortable to transform the discomfort into comfort. Here again, you have to give it up to get it. It is one thing to hear and understand the instruction of allowing discomfort to be present in your experience without doing anything about it. It's another thing, when you're in the relaxation session itself and there is discomfort, to remember and implement this instruction.

## The inner game of letting go: choosing to feel the refusal inside without having to change it at all

Throughout this section I am reiterating the point that accepting *what is* must necessarily and centrally include accepting all of the inner refusal, the inner kicking and screaming that says I don't want to accept *what is*, all aversion to accepting aversion—in short, all reactions in you that do not want to go along with the principle instructions that constitute *Paradoxical Relaxation.*

## No kidding

What I am describing here took me many years to understand. What I am describing is almost too subtle to be expressed in words. Yet it is the heart of the *Paradoxical Relaxation* method.

If you want to reap the benefit of *Paradoxical Relaxation*, it is important to understand the necessity of giving up trying to *make* some feeling or sensation comfortable when it is not comfortable. No kidding. You must find a way to *not* manipulate yourself into trying to change the uncomfortable into the comfortable. This means that you must earnestly and sincerely *choose* to find a way to accept what is uncomfortable in the moment.

In the moment of doing relaxation, one must release all hankering to feel better in order to feel better

You must be clear about what it means to choose to get as comfortable as you can with what is uncomfortable and tight and resists relaxation. This is a paradox. In order to transform discomfort into comfort, you really have to sincerely intend to accept the discomfort in the moment. You must inwardly renounce a more comfortable feeling inside you that is not there for you in the moment. In the moment of doing relaxation, there can be no hankering after feeling better if you want to feel better.

## Allowing discomfort to be an object in awareness instead of being merged in it

It is helpful when doing *Paradoxical Relaxation* to regard tension, discomfort, or pain as *objects* in awareness. When discomfort is an object in awareness, you have some distance from it and it is then possible to rest with it and accept it as it is. Imagine that when your attention is focused on your forehead you notice in the periphery of your awareness that you have a sense of impatience with lying down and keeping your attention continually focused on your forehead. That feeling of restlessness is a sensation and emotion that you are aware of inside yourself.

When you are *identified* with this restlessness and impatience, you make no distinction between who you are and these emotions-sensations. When you are merged with them and not separate from them, your impatience and restlessness are like carjackers who have taken over the steering wheel of your life. They control your attention and what you do. In being merged with restlessness and impatience, you do what these reactions inside you want you to do, which is to try to escape, distract yourself, space out, or leave the situation.

## Relaxation cannot occur when you are merged with impatience and restlessness

When emotions or sensations like restlessness and impatience become objects in awareness, you feel them but somehow are not merged inside of them. In experiencing restlessness and impatience as objects in awareness, you have stepped outside of them and are able to free yourself from their control over your attention. When you step outside of them, you become the subject and what you are aware of is the object. These emotions exist and you are a witness to them, but you are bigger than them. They exist in you, you don't exist within them. When you find that you contain them, you are not lost inside of them, you rest in them. In saying all of this, I reiterate that these emotions and resistances are part of us that we work to tame in the way I am describing in this book.

# Chapter 12

## *Preparation and logistics*

## Practical preparations and sequence in the practice of *Paradoxical Relaxation*

Logistics, with regard to relaxation, have to do with all of the circumstances and the environment (physical and psychological) around which you do relaxation. It has to do with the context in which your relaxation practice occurs: when you do it, where you do it, the clothes you wear, whether you go to the bathroom or not beforehand, etc.

Logistics are about creating an environment that is optimal for relaxation. It is not a good idea to do relaxation while watching television or otherwise being distracted.

## *Paradoxical Relaxation* preparation

The preparation for doing *Paradoxical Relaxation* is essential for its effectiveness. I encourage patients not to be disturbed for the period of time that they are doing the relaxation. This might mean asking their spouse to make sure that their children don't come into the room in which they are relaxing. I suggest too, if possible, that you disconnect the telephone and turn off the television or stereo. Relaxation needs to be done with no distractions, but it is most important to do it, even if the circumstances aren't ideal.

When possible, I tell patients to do their relaxation practice at a time when they do not have an important appointment immediately afterwards that requires them to be alert and tense. I suggest patients are alone in a chosen room, undisturbed by pets or other distractions.

## Using a timer

I have found that it is best to set a timer that will ring at the end of the relaxation session. When someone falls asleep during the relaxation period, the timer will indicate that the period is over. Because the relaxation is done first lying down, I advise the use of a pillow or two under the knees as a way of reducing stress on the lower back.

If patients have many things on their minds that preoccupy them in the relaxation session, it is a good idea to write them down on a piece of paper so that they will have less of a tendency to carry them in their head during relaxation. Also, I have found it is good to have a paper and pencil nearby while doing the relaxation. If a pressing thought arises, it can be jotted down and relaxation can be continued.

## Relaxation, eating, drinking, and the bathroom

It is best not to eat any substantial amount of food prior to relaxation as it tends to make one fall asleep. While falling asleep is not bad, it is better to remain awake throughout the entire relaxation session. Furthermore, I advise patients to avoid caffeine, sugar, or other stimulants prior to relaxation.

*In order to remain as comfortable as possible during the relaxation, I advise people to go to the bathroom if necessary before a period of relaxation.* It's best to avoid drinking fluids immediately prior to relaxation. Finally, most patients are more comfortable when they remove their glasses, loosen their tie, belt, or anything constricting.

## Setting up the room

I advise patients to partially darken the room in which they are going to relax and to use an eye pillow. An eye pillow is a small sack, often made of velvet or cotton and filled with flax seed or rice that can be bought at a health food store. It has the advantage of darkening the field of vision even in a room with a great deal of light. The eye pillow also tends to be soothing to the eyes and is usually helpful for relaxation.

*Paradoxical Relaxation* can be done lying down or in a chair. At the beginning of training, it is advised that it be done lying down with the knees bent but not resting on each other, especially if there is increased pain while sitting. A bed, a couch, a futon, or a carpeted floor will work. Sometimes patients are more comfortable lying on their side with a pillow between their knees even though this may tend to promote falling asleep. Because the key is comfort, it is acceptable to use as many pillows as necessary.

While it is good to have a comfortable regular place for relaxation, the practice can be done almost anywhere. It is possible to do *Paradoxical Relaxation* in a hotel room, on a bus, in a plane, in an office chair, in a park on the grass, or on a towel in the sand.

## What about falling asleep?

It is not uncommon to fall asleep during *Paradoxical Relaxation.* Falling asleep is more likely if you are tired and if you do the relaxation during a part of the day when you tend to become fatigued, such as the afternoon or evening.

*Paradoxical Relaxation* is not taking a nap. It is not uncommon, however, to fall asleep, especially if one is sleep deprived or taking sedating medication. Falling asleep is of little concern, especially in the beginning of relaxation training. It is preferable to doze rather than to tense for the purpose of staying awake. The experience of sleep during *Paradoxical Relaxation* tends to be different and usually more beneficial than simply falling asleep at night. When patients seem unable to remain awake during relaxation, I suggest that, if possible, they sit up and make sure the room is not overly warm.

## Emotional upset

Sometimes emotional upsets occur in our life. We have a fight with a friend or acquaintance, we get a letter from the IRS, we lose our wallet, we find out our job is in jeopardy. In this case, if possible, it's probably best to process the upset before doing relaxation. This includes talking to someone about it, making arrangements to solve the problem, or making a to-do list to at least organize your plan to deal with what has arisen. Once you've done everything that you can do for dealing with the problem that has arisen in your life, then you can do the relaxation even with the lingering distractions and the anxiety that you have. But as long as there's something that has to be done and the mind is not letting you rest until it is done, it's probably better to deal with the issue and then do the relaxation.

## The best time to do *Paradoxical Relaxation* is when you have the most energy

*The best time to do Paradoxical Relaxation is when you have the most energy.* Most people find that they have this kind of energy in the morning. However, this is not universally true. Some people have more energy and ability to pay attention in the afternoon.

*Paradoxical Relaxation* requires energy because this practice is attempting to modify a habit of inner tension that has been practiced countless times. Establishing a new habit in the face of such a practiced habit is very ambitious. It is for this reason that each practice period must 'really count' by virtue of the earnestness and level of attention with which it is done.

It is best to get into a routine of doing *Paradoxical Relaxation* so the body gets used to a regular time of quiet. A routine also helps avoid missing relaxation sessions. While I normally advise people to do *Paradoxical Relaxation* at least once a day, when possible it is preferable to do it twice a day. The best times tend to be in the morning and afternoon or evening, but before a major meal.

## The 10-20 minute rule of fussing: accepting the inevitable period of fussing and distraction that usually occurs in the beginning of the relaxation session

There is often a period of discomfort at the start of each relaxation session that you must go through if you are to learn relaxation. If you don't know how to persevere through it and get past it, you can become discouraged and give up. Therefore, how people deal with this period often determines how successful they become with *Paradoxical Relaxation*. Here is an example to illustrate the principle.

People who enjoy getting into a hot tub or hot bath know that there is a moment of discomfort as they slip into the water. This discomfort is due to the fact that their bodies are not acclimated to the heat and the heat feels almost oppressive or painful. If this initial feeling of heat didn't change, they couldn't stay in the hot water. However, they have learned that, after a few brief moments, their bodies acclimate to the temperature and the hot water becomes relaxing and pleasurable. The brief yet extreme initial discomfort ceases to be oppressive and soon becomes very comfortable.

If they were put off by this initial discomfort and were not willing to momentarily endure it in order to acclimate to it, they could never enjoy the benefits of the hot water.

I think it is helpful to consciously be aware of the fussing period that exists as you begin relaxation and the often subtle discomfort and struggle in focusing attention during that time. I found that when I expected that my relaxation would be immediate, and not fussy and uncomfortable at first, it took longer for me to quiet down.

Therefore, I think it is useful to accept this transition period in all of its dimensions. It is useful to completely accept that it takes some time for attention to focus, for the body to settle, for breathing to slow down, and generally for one to leave the state of activity for the state of being. This is a particular application of the idea discussed later of accepting everything that is going on inside you, exactly as it is, without any expectation that it be any different.

## What happens if you miss a session or fall off the wagon?

We are all human. In our treatment of pelvic pain,1` we have dealt with many patients who refused to do the relaxation at all because they hated the process of being still and addressing what was going on inside themselves. However, most patients in this category come around after awhile and realize that relaxation is an essential key to any recovery.

This process of abandoning the relaxation protocol for awhile and then coming back to it again is not abnormal. I have seen many patients succeed with their *Paradoxical Relaxation* regimen after they return to its daily practice.

That's one issue. Another issue is, what do you do if you miss a session? I think it is very important to be practicing relaxation every day, ideally twice a day; once in the morning, once in the evening. If you miss a session, of course, you just pick it up and get on it and do it again.

## Two relaxation sessions per day is ideal

To be effective, *Paradoxical Relaxation* needs to be done daily. While of course there will be some days it is not possible, missing relaxation should be the rare exception rather than the rule. As you become skilled in relaxation and it becomes part of your balance in life, you won't want to miss it. Effective *Paradoxical Relaxation* requires at least one half hour to one hour daily. This is often not easy with the demands of work, family and all the other circumstances of life.

# Chapter 13

## *Medication and other considerations*

## The role of medication in anxiety and tension disorders

In recent years, medications have increasingly become more and more prescribed for anxiety, depression, and related disorders. Almost everyone taking medications whom I have seen in my work with anxiety-related disorders would prefer to get off of them. In recent years, some mental health professionals have begun to consider it negligence to not offer the medication therapy route in dealing with anxiety. The idea here is that medication should be a component of most treatment plans for anxiety. This is a very perplexing idea to those of us who have never dealt with our anxiety through the use of medications.

While no one wants to rely on medications to control their moods, anxiety and related disorders can be hugely distressing to the point of being intolerable and medications may be necessary in the short term to manage the intolerable distress of some individuals who are anxious. The aim of *Paradoxical Relaxation* is to offer a better treatment for anxiety than drug treatment. In fact, one of the aims of *Paradoxical Relaxation* in selected people is to essentially replace the use of drugs as the primary method of reducing or stopping anxiety.

## Medications that are skillfully used are a blessing

It is important to say that it is easy to demonize medications and I want to appreciate that they exist and are as helpful as they are. Medications for anxiety used skillfully are a blessing. The problem with medication occurs when it is thoughtlessly prescribed as a matter of convenience for the doctor who has 15 minutes to get on to the next patient.

In my work with people who have pelvic pain, the question has often arisen as to whether they should continue using medication in learning the *Wise-Anderson Protocol*. It has happened more than once that someone has come to one of our clinics with the idea that they did not want to use medication once they started our protocol. Typically, a day or two later, their pain and/or anxiety for which they had been taking the medication, rebounded.

I generally don't think it is a good idea for people to stop taking medications for anxiety that they have been relying on when first starting *Paradoxical Relaxation* training until they have developed some skill in the method as I discuss below. And a reduction in medication should be done with the supervision of a physician.

## The downside of using medications

The issue of using medications for anxiety is not simple. Medications are often helpful in reducing anxiety, pain, and depressive symptoms. These benefits, however, don't come without a price, and in some cases, a big price.

*When you use medication, you tend to learn little about how to deal with your symptoms other than through the use of the medication.* It is easy to take medication. You pop it into your mouth and you wait for the effect or you take it regularly to maintain a certain blood level of the drug that permits whatever effect the drug has to continue. Though not true for everyone, I believe that in general, using the medications tends to reduce the motivation to learn a non-drug way to help reduce or stop anxiety.

## The side effects of medication

Medications come with numerous side effects. Addiction is often a major problem and this is true in particular of the benzodiazepines. Certain antidepressants used for the control of anxiety can paradoxically exacerbate anxiety.

In addition, there can be side effects such as mental fogginess, lethargy, depression, and increased anxiety between doses which can be the result of inter-dose withdrawal.

Typically, over time, medications become less effective at the initial dosage levels, and it often becomes necessary to increase the dosage and frequency of use in order for the medications to have the same effect on symptoms.

## A major goal of *Paradoxical Relaxation* is to help patients become free of the need for medication

Most everyone who is interested in learning Paradoxical Relaxation does not want to use medication. A goal of *Paradoxical Relaxation* is to remove the necessity of using medications on any regular basis. It is generally agreed that stopping the use of psychotropic medications suddenly is a bad idea. I think it makes much more sense to continue the use of the medications for anxiety, under physician supervision, through the initial training in *Paradoxical Relaxation* until your skill might allow you to begin to reduce your anxiety or other symptoms using the method.

Once you become skillful at *Paradoxical Relaxation*, you may be able to reduce your symptoms reliably beyond where your medications typically reduce them. In coming off of medications while learning *Paradoxical* Relaxation, most physicians who are consulted understand that medication for anxiety must be reduced very slowly so that there should be no 'cold turkey' experimentation. This is particularly true of the benzodiazepines and opiates. Coming off of drugs, and substituting relaxation and cognitive therapy as the major anti-anxiety strategies, needs to be done with a doctor's supervision.

In summary, medications used skillfully can be of great help. Other than in certain rare circumstances, however, the use of medications on a long-term basis for dealing with anxiety and anxiety-related disorders is not my preference. I think of *Paradoxical Relaxation* as a *non-drug anti-anxiety strategy*, a substitute for medications that reduces or stops anxiety without side-effects and continues to increase in efficacy with practice.

# What helps *Paradoxical Relaxation* training

## Hot baths before relaxation or myofascial release

Hot baths, sauna, or other ways of warming the body are an underrated assistance in calming down anxiety and anxiety-related disorders. A hot bath doesn't work for everyone, but can be effective in lowering nervous system arousal by itself. A hot bath, shower, or sauna is particularly effective in preparing the body for *Paradoxical Relaxation.* Using heat to help reduce nervous arousal and prepare the body for the methods described in this book has few side effects and is readily available and inexpensive. If heat is helpful for your anxiety, accessibility to a hot tub is usually a good idea.

## Giving up addiction to the news

When you are in a chronically anxious state, you tend to be hypersensitive to disturbing news and images. Yet, we are living in a world now where disturbing news and images can inundate us from a number of venues that did not exist 20 years ago. In just going online and looking at your default homepage, you will typically encounter all kinds of news, often involving bad news, and disturbing images that often are agitating.

In dealing with my own tendency toward anxiety, I gave up having television 20 years ago. In a way, it was like weaning myself off of an addictive drug. My normal lifestyle would involve coming home and turning on the television. In the home I grew up in, my father would turn the television on as soon as he woke up and it would be on whenever we were home. We lived in the kitchen and of course there was a television in there.

## Giving up television

I found that in giving up television in my life, my nervous system tended to quiet down. I had to get used to not having the distraction of television when I would come home. After several months of television-free living I came to appreciate the lack of disturbance that was the benefit of not having television. For the chronically anxious person, I recommend a trial of no television. Removing television for 3 or 4 months (you have to give yourself a few months to get used to life without television) can allow you to see if such a choice helps you calm down.

I am not suggesting that you hide your head in the sand and never listen to any current events. In all of the 20 or so years that I have gone without television, the news that I needed to know about seems to easily have found its way to me. I feel my life has been enhanced by removing television from my home and the compulsive need to be up to the minute with current events. Pico Iyer wrote an illuminating essay in the *New York Times* in which he said, regarding giving up the 24/7 news cycle in contemporary media, "…the 24/7 news cycle has propelled people up and down and down and up and then left them pretty much where they started."

## Taking a long view: managing your expectations

Unrealistic expectations of Paradoxical Relaxation will make you anxious and increase your pain and suffering. In my view, anxiety and anxiety-related disorders do not come about out of the blue, even though in some cases it may seem so. It is said that the fruit falls suddenly from the tree even though the ripening takes a long time. It is my view that someone can have chronic anxiety for years without symptoms and then with age or certain stresses the symptoms are triggered. Just as anxiety symptoms don't spontaneously appear, neither do they disappear overnight. In my experience, even with our most successful patients, symptoms take a significant amount of time to resolve.

I suggest that patients who begin *Paradoxical Relaxation* give themselves 3-6 months in which to practice it before expecting symptoms to begin to become reliably better. For those who are helped by this relaxation protocol, symptoms usually continue to improve (although flare-ups are common with stressful events) as people practice our methodology over time. Of course, not everyone benefits from *Paradoxical Relaxation*, but for those who do, it usually takes a considerable period of time for symptoms to reliably quiet down.

### Evaluating your progress after 3-6 months does not mean that you won't have periods of feeling better soon after beginning practice

*Taking 3-6 months before you evaluate the effect of Paradoxical Relaxation does not mean that you will not experience a benefit quite soon after beginning treatment.* Giving yourself this period of time means understanding that typically a person's condition fluctuates, especially at the beginning of treatment.

### The wisdom of not celebrating when you are feeling better, or despairing when you are feeling worse

I suggest that patients resist celebrating when they are feeling better, or despairing when they are feeling worse. Typically during the practice of paradoxical relaxation, patients can have many flare-ups of anxiety and related symptoms, often followed by an improvement.

I have touched on the challenge of resting the nervous system and having the need to use it to function in life. In an ideal world, we would send our nervous system to a tropical island for a long rest. Unfortunately, this is not possible. We cannot avoid the stresses and strains of daily life that interfere with the calming down of our nervous system and our nervous system's 'idle speed.'

## Moment-to-Moment Relaxation

### *Moment-to-Moment Relaxation* in a nutshell

*Moment-to-Moment Relaxation* is the practice of continuously letting go of slight tensions that build up moment to moment throughout the day. Especially when you are anxious, certain default sites of tension remain continually tensed, and allowing them to relax as much as they can usually only occurs for the brief period of time your attention is on the tension. As soon as you take your attention off of the habitually contracted part of your body, it will typically tighten right back up. It is for this reason that the instruction of *Moment-to-Moment Relaxation* is to go back and let go of the re-tensed up part of the body over and over again. Doing *Moment-to-Moment Relaxation* all day can sometimes have a significant lowering on the idle speed of the nervous system.

> Moment-to-Moment Relaxation is the practice of continuously letting go of slight tensions that build up moment by moment throughout the day

When doing *Moment-to-Moment Relaxation*, don't look for immediate results. Don't strain in any way. It should just take a moment to notice the tension and do *Moment-to-Moment Relaxation*. Remember that your voluntary relaxation of these muscles at first will rarely cause much of a sense of relaxation in them. Even if this method is effective for you, you may not experience any relief of symptoms for days or weeks. Nevertheless, it is important to do this relaxation on an ongoing basis until it becomes a habit that replaces the tendency of chronically tightening the tensed part of the body.

Patients are often surprised at the number of times each day that they find themselves all tensed up. The places in the body that bear the brunt of this tension may be the forehead, eyes, face, neck, shoulders, arms, hands, chest, back, belly, pelvis, and legs. Changing the habit of tightening up these places is not a small matter.

## ***Moment-to-Moment Relaxation*** **is used throughout your normal day to regularly interrupt the habit of continuously contracting your body**

In the *Wise-Anderson Protocol* for pelvic pain, we use *Paradoxical Relaxation* in two different but complementary ways. *Moment-to-Moment Relaxation* is used throughout your normal day to regularly interrupt the habit of tensing muscles that tend to be continually contracted. Doing *Moment-to-Moment Relaxation* therefore can involve many tiny relaxations during the day. As you become more skilled, this practice takes less time and is done almost automatically. The intention here is for you to abort the old, dysfunctional chronic habits of tensing certain places in your body.

*Moment-to-Moment Relaxation* does not offer the depth of relaxation achieved by *Paradoxical Relaxation, but* can have clear though limited effects. The intensive practice of *Paradoxical Relaxation* represents the laboratory in which the skill of the method is developed. It represents the heart of the practice and produces the most benefit. The skill of feeling, accepting, and resting with tension that can *make it possible for anxiety to reduce or disappear, is honed in the Paradoxical Relaxation* practice.

In doing *Moment-to-Moment Relaxation*, it is sometimes useful to use a small and inexpensive device called *The MotivAider.* Recently, certain vibration watches have come on the market that can be set to vibrate for certain set periods of time as well. These devices vibrate silently and repeatedly like someone tapping you on the shoulder at times you designate, to remind you to let go of any tension you might be unnecessarily holding in your body. For instance, you can set one of these devices to vibrate every ten minutes, or every hour, as a private reminder to relax the part of the body you wish to particularly relax like the shoulders, neck, jaw, or pelvic muscles.

## ***Moment-to-Moment Relaxation* practice is aimed at subtracting tension from habitual tension throughout the day**

*Moment-to-Moment Paradoxical Relaxation* is like using a thimble to empty water in a row boat. Occasionally the effect of doing this upon symptoms is dramatic; usually it is not. *I tell patients to continue to do it whether you have results or not.*

Practicing this hundreds of times for several weeks, for instance, has helped some patients with anxiety issues significantly reduce their symptoms. You have to be motivated, however, to come out of the unconscious swoon most people are in during the day in order to pay attention to and release yourself from the chronic guarding.

*Moment-to-Moment Relaxation* can similarly help reduce symptoms in stress related disorders like pelvic pain, headache, bruxism and jaw pain, shoulder, and neck pain among others. Some individuals experience no benefit from doing this practice. Although quite unusual, when we published the first edition of our book *A Headache in the Pelvis*, one man said doing *Moment-to-Moment Relaxation* for several months reduced his symptoms by 90%.

## Hints on the application of the *Moment-to-Moment Relaxation*

1. **It takes time to learn**

It takes time to learn how to do *Moment-to-Moment Relaxation* so that it does not interrupt your day. Doing it should take only a moment or two.

2. **Make sure that you do not exert effort**

Make sure you do not exert any effort to relax. This kind of relaxation is just a simple letting go of tension that *easily* relaxes. It must not feel hard or difficult or straining in any way. It should feel easy just like lifting up your arm and then letting it drop. As soon as you feel tension that is not easily relaxed, make no further efforts.

3. **Continue to practice even if no results seem to occur**

*Moment-to-Moment* relaxation subtracts tension from the default tension level people live with on a moment to moment basis. Typically there is little or no benefit felt with each particular momentary letting go. The benefit of *Moment-to-Moment Relaxation* is cumulative and is felt in the back-end rather than the front-end of this practice. For this reason, it is best to have no expectation of results on a moment to moment basis.

# Chapter 14

## *Paradoxical Relaxation* for an *anxiety state*

## The *anxiety state*

There is a state that many people enter at some time in their life that can be called an *anxiety state*. The *anxiety state* is different from everyday anxiety. When you are in an *anxiety state*, the nervous system doesn't seem to calm down and the kind of relief and ability to relax that occurs when anxieties come and go are few and far between. An *anxiety state* feels awful and traditionally has been difficult to treat. In recent times, medications have tended to be quickly prescribed, although their efficacy is mixed. I want to discuss the place of *Paradoxical Relaxation* in helping someone to come out of an *anxiety state*.

> If you were to take a snapshot of the state of your body and mind during a momentary period of worry, the anxiety state would be an ongoing caricature of that state

## Anxiety is a fancy word for fear

The word anxiety has been traced to 1624, from the Latin word *anxius*, meaning troubled in mind. It is also traced back to the Latin word *angere* meaning to cause distress. Today, anxiety is a 'fancy' word for fear. It is also used to describe what is called nervousness, jumpiness, being stressed out, freaked out, panicked, worried, concerned, and fretting. These are all synonyms for anxiety.

Anxiety is a normal biological reaction to a situation in which you feel some kind of threat. I have described Walter Cannon's work discussing the varieties of survival responses in his typology of *fight, flight, freeze*. These responses are clearly appropriate in the face of something that truly is a threat to your survival. We all deal with fear because we are vulnerable organisms in a world that carries many dangers, health, and well-being. Anxiety becomes a problem when its presence in your life is the rule rather than the exception and is inappropriately elicited by things about which you fret and worry that objectively harbor little real danger.

## The *anxiety state* occurs when nervous system arousal goes over the *redline*

In chapter two, I discussed the *upregulated nervous system* and the idle speed of a car engine. On a graph that measures nervous system arousal, I discussed the various positions someone can be in, relative to the symptom threshold and explained why some people can become anxious with very little provocation and some people can remain anxiety-free with apparently a great deal of provocation.

The *anxiety state* can also be understood using another automotive metaphor of the tachometer in a car that measures the speed of rotation of the car engine. The speed of a car engine's rotation is a measure of how hard the engine is working.

The tachometer's display contains a section called the *redline.* The purpose of the *redline* is to indicate to the driver that the engine is being run faster than designed and it can be damaged if the car continues to be run at such speed.

If you run a car at speeds over the redline for ongoing periods of time, all kinds of difficulties can follow. The engine can overheat, the bearings can fail, the brakes can wear out quickly, the fatigue limits of the metal, pistons and heads can be exceeded, and the car can become unstable. The engine isn't designed to be run at redline speeds for any prolonged period of time.

## The *anxiety state* occurs when the nervous system is going too fast for too long

The *anxiety state* can be understood to occur when the speed or activity of the nervous system is significantly heightened. The redline of the nervous system can be thought to be that level of nervous system arousal that, when maintained chronically, results in a number of distressing symptoms.

When the anxiety or fear state goes on too long and is too strong, a person can experience a variety of bewildering symptoms that I list later in this chapter. When the nervous system reaches a certain chronic level of arousal, the slightest little thing triggers someone's catastrophic thinking and fearful projection into the future. *Negative thoughts can feel like blows in the anxiety state.*

I have had several episodes in my life of being in an *anxiety state* so I know it from personal experience as well as having treated many patients. The *anxiety state*s I experienced lasted for a number of months and were very scary and distressing. In my life, they were related to major life events like the death of a relative or a relationship ending.

## Panic Disorder

When you are in an *anxiety state*, there is a special kind of very intense, very painful spike in nervous system arousal called the panic attack. Panic attacks occur when the level of arousal crosses high above the *redline* of the nervous system. In such a state, you feel that you can't tolerate being in your own skin because the feeling of panic is overwhelming. Once someone has a panic attack, he or she often goes around worrying about having another attack and the thought itself of having a panic attack becomes a major stressor.

## The *anxiety state* is a certain altered state like the state that occurs with intoxication

When I found myself in an *anxiety state*, I had the sense that my biochemistry was somehow altered from its normal state. I felt that I had lost my balance in the same way as I could lose my balance and sense of proportion if I had too much to drink

When I was in an *anxiety state*, I felt like I could not stop my anxiety even when the situation was resolved. It felt like the floor of my emotional stability fell out from under me. Tiny stresses frightened me. I couldn't sleep. I couldn't control my catastrophic thinking. I worried about my health. I worried about those I loved. I worried about whether I was going to be able to take care of myself. I couldn't rest or calm down. I couldn't relax.

In the *anxiety state*, I felt that I was in a changed state inside, that the re-orienting and resetting of my nervous system that normally occurred after sleep, rest, and other rejuvenating activities was impaired. If I was normally upset about something, after a night of sleep I woke up and felt much better and more able to handle the problem. In the *anxiety state*, my anxiety and worry didn't seem to get better the next day… it endured day after day. I know that my tendency toward anxiety is what underlay my pelvic pain. It was my suffering with anxiety and pelvic pain that forced me to find a way to deal with them. This suffering is what prompted me to learn what I now call *Paradoxical Relaxation.*

Just as the list is very long as to how the ability to deeply relax is beneficial, so the list is very long as to how the *anxiety state* can feel so debilitating. While time and space do not permit any comprehensive discussion of the profoundly distressing effects of the *anxiety state*, I will touch on these effects below.

## Anxiety interferes with our ability to think

The *anxiety state* makes learning, comprehension, and holding information difficult. We learn best when we are relaxed and untroubled. If you remember being particularly anxious, you'll remember how difficult it was to focus your attention. When you're chronically anxious, sometimes you tend to deal with the anxiety by being fastidious and over-organized. More often than not, however, in such a state your ability to organize and keep things organized becomes compromised. In the *anxiety state*, inhibiting emotions and impulses tends to be more difficult. When we are in an *anxiety state,* we tend to do and say things that in a calmer state we wouldn't consider saying or doing.

When someone is in the *anxiety state,* his or her attention tends to compulsively return to what they are anxious about. This also occurs during relaxation. One of the challenges of relaxing while anxious is gaining control over attention that is even more distracted.

The *anxiety state* often prompts disturbances in eating. It is not uncommon for someone to lose their appetite. Compulsive eating or compulsive dieting are related to the *anxiety state.* Anorexia and bulimia are typically associated with anxiety.

The *anxiety state* is almost always associated with sleep disturbances. Difficulty falling asleep and staying asleep are frequent consequences. Occasionally sleeping too much is one way some people cope in the *anxiety state,* but more commonly insomnia occurs in states of anxiety. Sleep deprivation tends to exacerbate the *problem* and tends to compromise the ability to retain information in the short-term, to pay attention, and to do a task well.

## Compulsive behaviors that attempt to reduce anxiety often create more problems

I have seen an *anxiety state* lead to behaviors that attempt to reduce anxiety but ultimately create more problems. For instance, the *anxiety state* can be associated with what is called 'workaholism' which is a tendency to work compulsively to escape from or distract oneself from anxiety. The *anxiety state* can be connected to compulsive drug and alcohol abuse. Addiction to these substances often becomes the main problem when they are used for the self-medication of anxiety, masking the anxiety that still has to be dealt with when the addictive behavior is brought under control.

## Anxiety and creativity

In the *anxiety state,* creativity is typically difficult. While it is true that some people flee to creativity to escape anxiety, more often than not, intense anxiety makes being creative and playful much more difficult. The *anxiety state* is not a good muse. Mozart is reputed to have complained about how difficult it was for him to write music when he was chronically worried about paying the rent and struggling with other financial difficulties.

## Anxiety and interpersonal relationships

In the *anxiety state,* close relationships typically tend to be strained. You tend to be preoccupied and not present with other people as well as being short, irritable, withdrawn, dismissive, inconsiderate, and less skillful interpersonally. Irritability with, resentment of, or over-dependency on others is common.

The *anxiety state* is easily felt by others. When someone is in an *anxiety state,* others can feel the anxiety exuding from them and it can be agitating just to be around them. The person or people close to those in an *anxiety state* often have a difficult time being with them.

## Symptoms associated with the *anxiety state*

While I will be discussing the symptoms of specific disorders related to anxiety in the following sections, anxiety states can be accompanied by these feelings and physical symptoms:

- Increased nervousness
- Feeling of butterflies in the stomach
- Hyperactivity or hypoactivity of gastrointestinal tract
- Libido is reduced
- Increased sweating in the palms and elsewhere
- Increased heart rate and blood pressure
- Jumpiness, twitching, fidgeting
- Headache
- Clammy hands, sweating, dry mouth
- Depression
- Rapid heartbeat
- Headache
- Nausea

- Trembling/tremor
- Loss or increase in appetite
- Difficulty concentrating
- Dry mouth
- Panic
- Muscle tension, nervous irritability
- Discomfort of the gastrointestinal tract, including constipation and/or diarrhea
- Distractibility
- Sleep disturbance including difficulty falling or staying asleep
- Dizziness/light headedness
- Uncontrollable, often irrational, compulsive worry

## Using *Paradoxical Relaxation* to help resolve an *anxiety state*

The *anxiety state* can be likened to the elephant in the story of the elephant and the blind man discussed earlier. The phenomenon of anxiety has different sides. In the simple breakdown, there are the experiential, physiological, behavioral, and mental sides of anxiety.

In the experiential side of the *anxiety state,* you can feel tense, agitated, frightened, hyper-vigilant, or tired. You can't seem to concentrate, very little is enjoyable, the future looks bleak, and your self-esteem is typically low. You can't enjoy anything. This is the subjective, experiential side of the *anxiety state.*

*Then there is the physiological side of the anxiety state.* The blood pressure and heart rate of the anxious person tend to be elevated, salivation is inhibited and the mouth is dry, the sweat response increases, blood drains from the periphery and the hands become clammy and cold, muscle tension increases, hyperactivity or hypoactivity of the gastrointestinal tract occurs, libido reduces, sleep is disturbed, ability to concentrate is reduced as the amygdala of the brain is activated which bombards and interferes with functioning of the cerebral cortex (the part of the brain necessary to think rationally), and there are many other physiological signs of a frightened animal.

*There is the behavioral side of the anxiety state.* Without any modification or intervention, the anxious person can be irritable or withdrawn from interpersonal relationships, can make impulsive decisions, can continually view situations pessimistically and act accordingly, can function poorly at work or in situations that require focus and the ability to think, and can generally act out from the fearful views that he holds of the world.

*There is the mental side of the anxiety state.* As I have discussed, the thinking of someone who is in an *anxiety state* tends to be negative and catastrophic, picturing the worst case scenario in many situations. They usually have a poor ability to pay attention. When you ask a person in an *anxiety state* to focus on sensation, as we do in *Paradoxical Relaxation*, at first attention can only be held for a few seconds before attention is distracted. Attention in the *anxiety state* is like the attention of a bird, continually flitting from one thing to another as he scans the environment for danger.

The person in an *anxiety state* lives like Damocles in the $4^{th}$ century Greek legend. Damocles was condemned to live under a sharpened sword that was hung from heaven by a single horse hair. Damocles never knew when the horse hair would break and so lived with the threat of disaster each moment as the thin hair offered no assurance that in the next moment it would continue to hold up the sword. The Roman orator Cicero used the story of Damocles to make the insightful observation about the anxious human being that *there can be nothing happy for the person over whom some fear always looms.*

*The treatment of the anxiety state that I am proposing, of which Paradoxical Relaxation is one the central methods, aims to intervene on all of these different dimensions—experiential, physiological, behavioral, and mental.*

## The antidote to the *anxiety state*: cultivating the mindset and inner physical posture of someone who is peaceful

We normally think about peace of mind as a lofty and ongoing state of the old and the wise. Peace of mind means a quiet mind with no thoughts. Peace of mind allows you to relax and allows your emergency center to put the 'all clear' message out. Peace of mind has no need for adrenaline and other stress response hormones in your blood stream.

When you are practicing *Paradoxical Relaxation*, you are practicing resting in the mindset of someone who is at peace inside. In *Paradoxical Relaxation,* you practice not paying attention to thought. Every time your attention is distracted by a thought, the *Paradoxical Relaxation* instruction is to return attention to sensation without attending to the thought. In *Paradoxical Relaxation,* you practice ignoring thoughts that arise in the mind whether positive or negative. In this way, you step out of the symbolic world created by your thinking.

This basic instruction in *Paradoxical Relaxation* is particularly challenging when you are in an *anxiety state.* In the *anxiety state,* there is typically a heightened wariness about letting go of thought because thinking is the way somebody in an *anxiety state* remains vigilant. For this reason, it is particularly important for people in an *anxiety state* to be in the presence of a teacher whom they trust. The trusted teacher will tend to routinely reassure the patient that it is safe to let go of thinking and rest attention in sensation.

The wariness about taking attention away from vigilant thinking is just one of the particular obstacles of doing *Paradoxical Relaxation* in an *anxiety state.* When you are in an *anxiety state,* you can become much more easily frightened about thoughts and feelings that occur inside you. In the beginning of training, the reassurance of the teacher of *Paradoxical Relaxation* can be like a life preserver for someone who is in the water and can't swim.

## Peace of mind means no thinking

The engine of the *anxiety state* is uncontrollable worry and catastrophic thinking. When I was in an *anxiety state*, I worried about the symptoms I was having in the *anxiety state* and feared that they meant the worst for me. I had no ability to stop my anxious thinking.

It is possible to learn Paradoxical Relaxation
in the middle of an anxiety state

In the *anxiety state*, the main strategy I propose is both cognitive therapy and *Paradoxical Relaxation.* When you are in an *anxiety state*, if you are willing to persist in following the protocol despite what is uncomfortable, it is possible to succeed in calming down your nervous system.

## The practice of saying *yes* to a very loud *no* inside

In *Paradoxical Relaxation*, we practice assuming an attitude of inwardly saying *yes* to everything. In *Paradoxical Relaxation* we practice saying *yes* to the unconscious *no* inside, of which we seem to have little control. This *no* is palpably experienced inside as stubborn tension that does not release.

Practicing an attitude and viewpoint of *yes* is a great challenge to the very loud inner *no* of fear and contraction in the *anxiety state.* It is the practice of accepting everything in your experience as it is in the moment. This is the practice of non-resistance, non-clinging, non-attachment. Whatever is here in this moment is what we practice feeling and allow to exist without judgment or resistance.

It is the practice of allowing the inner refusal inside us to exist without being controlled by it. In the musical *Fiddler on the Roof,* two men bring a dispute that they are having in front of the rabbi. One man says, "It was a horse." The other man says, "It was a mule." To the first man, the rabbi says, "You're right." To the second man the rabbi turns and says, "You're right." A third observer says to the rabbi, "How can both of them be right?" To this third man the rabbi says, "You're right too." In *Paradoxical Relaxation,* all the constrictions, inner argument, discomforts, and resistances are all right. In honoring them all, you paradoxically facilitate their quickest resolution.

In doing *Paradoxical Relaxation*, when in the *anxiety state*, we practice the mental and physical discipline required to allow us not to judge or regard anything in our immediate experience as wrong. In the moment of *Paradoxical Relaxation*, we practice allowing to exist whatever is in our immediate experience whether or not we perceive it as uncomfortable. We practice feeling sensation inside of us without resisting any of it. This practice includes accepting the part of us that judges and resists what is unpleasant or fearful.

## The relief of bringing the attitude of acceptance into the *anxiety state*

The *anxiety state* is the state of emergency. It is the state in which the primitive organism is terrified. It is a state in which everything is not okay, not safe, fearful, and dangerous. In the *anxiety state,* we can easily become frightened by our own shadow.

When you enter into the *Paradoxical Relaxation* session, you are taking a position opposed by the *anxiety state* you are in. At first, anxiety may slightly increase as your body faces the challenge of letting down its guard. It is for this reason that it is best when no force or coercion be used. It only stalemates your inner resistance to try to force yourself to do anything or be any particular way.

When you begin to practice *Paradoxical Relaxation* in an *anxiety state*, it is important to go slowly and if necessary reduce the time of each session to a duration that is tolerable to you. If you find that you have difficulty lying still for a half-hour, it is advisable to reduce the time to 20 minutes and then work your way up to a half-hour.

When doing Paradoxical Relaxation in an anxiety state, it is particularly important to clearly understand that your fear is not your enemy

One of the major obstacles those in an *anxiety state* face when doing *Paradoxical Relaxation* is their own fear of their anxiety. For this reason, it is particularly important to understand that accepting fear in an *anxiety state* simply means noticing the sensations associated with fear and allowing them to be present without having to do anything about them. While there will typically be resistance to accepting the sensations of the fear, such acceptance will open the door to the anxiety dissolving.

## Anxiety and rope burns

It has been said that suffering is a rope burn. A rope burn occurs when we cling to the rope that won't allow us a firm grasp. The concept is that when we cling to anything, we suffer. This is because everything in life is transient and eventually we will lose it. In this metaphor, the rope burn represents everything to which we are attached or averse to—those things that we either want to keep in our life or keep out of our life. The opposite of the rope burn can be illustrated by the poem *Kiss the Joy as it Flies* by William Blake.

He who binds himself to joy
Does the winged life destroy
But he who kisses joy as it flies
Lives in eternity's sunrise.

William Blake

In *Paradoxical Relaxation*, during an *anxiety state*, we are kissing the contraction, sorrow, anxiety and the pain, in fact metaphorically everything in our experience as it flies in the moment. In doing *Paradoxical Relaxation in* an *anxiety state,* our focus is on *reorienting our reaction* to what goes on in our inner experience moment by moment.

Instead of waiting for our inner experience of contraction to change, we change our viewpoint toward our inner experience. Instead of waiting for the earth to be covered with leather to make walking comfortable, we put on leather shoes and then can walk anywhere comfortably. Instead of trying to change our experience in the moment to what we want it to be, we practice being okay with whatever is in our experience.

## Relaxing with everything as it is, is strong medicine for the *anxiety state*

The person who is peaceful inside accepts things as they are in the moment. In the moment of him being peaceful, he has no quarrel with the world.

A dear friend of mine told me a story that illustrates this principle. A number of years ago he was in a hopelessly crowded square in India. He said that in the space of a few acres, there could have been 20,000 people. Beggars, lepers, scrawny dogs and cats and chickens, oxen, pollution-spewing taxis, malnourished children, beautiful women in bright saris, smells of dung mingling with cooking food being prepared on the street—the space he was in was teeming with all the varieties of life.

My friend told me that at first he was disturbed by the scene. His mind was full of judgment. There were too many people, too much pollution, too much illness, too much poverty—too much of this and not enough of that. Then somehow in a moment of grace, in one of those rare epiphanies in life, his mind cleared and he felt overwhelmed with gratitude for everyone who was there. He told me that he came to feel that not one person was extraneous. There was not one person or one part of the scene that should not have been there and if one person was taken out or one aspect of the scene was modified, the whole of the scene would be violated.

He was overwhelmed with the desire to express his gratitude to everyone. Like a madman, to many perplexed looks, he went from person after person thanking them for being there. My friend's experience at that moment was the experience of being at peace—of saying *yes* to everything and of seeing and experiencing things as whole and complete exactly as they were. This experience did not come from a change in the situation itself, but from a shift in my friend's consciousness that allowed him to see the scene this way.

My friend said that he himself felt in a state of wholeness, lacking nothing, wanting nothing. Through just a shift of his viewpoint, hell became heaven; tension, resistance, and judgment became profound relaxation, and peace.

The kind of experience my friend had where there was apparently no effort involved in his overwhelming sense of gratitude, wholeness, and dissolution of all fear is rare. In *Paradoxical Relaxation,* we are engaging in a mental and physical discipline to enter such a state of wholeness and relaxation in which we exclude nothing. Excluding something from ourselves in the moment means tightening up against it. In *Paradoxical Relaxation*, we take attention away from thought and all else that is disturbing to our nervous system. In taking attention away from thinking, we don't tighten up against thoughts. Instead, we direct our attention to rest in sensation.

## In practicing *Paradoxical Relaxation* we practice an attitude and mental discipline to bring us into the mindset of the person who experiences no anxiety

The *anxiety state* is a state of *no*, a state of fear and vigilance. It is a state where you feel little control over your emotions. In practicing *Paradoxical Relaxation,* we practice an attitude and mental discipline to bring us into the mindset of the person who experiences no anxiety. We practice saying *yes* to everything in our experience including the part of us that can't say *yes* to everything. In becoming skilled in *Paradoxical Relaxation,* we can gain control over our emotions and our fear that feels so out of control in an *anxiety state.*

## Medications and an *anxiety state*

Medications are often prescribed for an *anxiety state* when simply reducing the symptoms of the *anxiety state* is the focus and there is no long-term strategy. The current medical model tends to be short-term, not unlike the way in which many politicians and corporate executives tend to look at political and economic issues and make decisions about them.

While medications can be important in temporarily managing the overwhelming intensity of symptoms in an *anxiety state*, medications used regularly over an extended period of time can be problematic. In my experience, medications alone rarely end the *anxiety state*. Medications given for an *anxiety state* tend to be used for a long period of time. Also, I have seen with a number of my patients, that along with helping to temporarily quiet the nervous system down, medications can cause problems of habituation or addiction to the drug. Sometimes, especially with the benzodiazepines, you can go through distressing withdrawal symptoms between doses.

When I was in an *anxiety state,* medications were not readily prescribed and I had to find other means to come back into balance. I don't believe that medication should *always* be used in an *anxiety state*, particularly if the patient does not want to use them. Of course, if the patient feels that the symptoms in the *anxiety state* are intolerable, if there is an issue of suicide or some other compelling reason, I believe that medications are certainly appropriate and important. But when patients express their desire to deal with their *anxiety state* without drugs and the doctor can give them tools to do so, I believe in supporting the patients in that desire to see if they can find a way to come out of the anxiety state without drugs. Men and women have gone in and come out of *anxiety states* throughout history without medications.

## The skillful use of drugs in panic disorder

When someone has been having panic attacks, it is often useful to carry a benzodiazepine as a sort of 'talisman' to ward off the panic attack. This is effective because often one of the worst parts of having panic attacks is the fear itself of having another attack. That fear of future attacks can be enough to bring one on. Carrying around a pill that you know within 30 minutes of taking will stop the panic attack, can help reduce the fear of the panic attack. That in itself is a therapy. It is sort of like having a life jacket close to you when you are swimming in deep water.

## It is possible to dig the well when the house is on fire: learning relaxation in the *anxiety state*

I have described the metaphor of digging a well when the house is on fire. This metaphor alludes to an emergency situation requiring immediate attention when what is needed is not immediately available. In the case of an *anxiety state*, the distressing symptoms call out for immediate relief and yet when you are first learning *Paradoxical Relaxation,* beginner's skill is not developed enough to offer you much relief. It takes a number of hours of relaxation practice to gain the slightest ability to reduce the arousal of your nervous system. Just as it is better to have the well dug so the water is immediately available to put out the fire, so it is that it would be better to be skillful in *Paradoxical Relaxation* to be able to immediately calm down the heightened nervous system arousal associated with the *anxiety state.* Nevertheless it is possible to dig the well even when the house is on fire.

When you are not practiced in *Paradoxical Relaxation* and you are in an *anxiety state*, it can take time for *Paradoxical Relaxation* to help you have a chance to begin to get relief from your anxiety. Being in an *anxiety state* is always scary because you've lost your balance and you don't know how to get it back. Patience is not the strong suit of the *anxiety state.*

Being in an *anxiety state* is not very different from being in chronic pain. Like chronic pain, when you are in an *anxiety state*, it is hard to imagine that you ever will be out of it. Sometimes it feels like you have no skin that separates you from the world—and everything in the world affects you directly. It is kind of like having a car with no shock absorbers and every single little bump reverberates in your bones. Lying down and doing *Paradoxical Relaxation* at first can be quite scary because you are lying down with what, typically, you just want to run away from. Everything that I talk about in doing *Paradoxical Relaxation* in terms of obstacles one can face is magnified when you are in an *anxiety state.*

It is important to learn relaxation with the help of someone who is not afraid of your *anxiety state* and somebody who can reassure you that it is okay to allow yourself to feel fear and discomfort and permit them both to be present. What you can learn about managing anxiety and managing your mind can serve you for the rest of your life.

# Chapter 15

## *Paradoxical Relaxation for anxiety-related disorders*

## ***Paradoxical Relaxation* and the treatment of functional disorders**

A functional disorder is a disorder of physiological functioning with no outstanding, organic structural pathology to account for symptoms. When you have a functional disorder in your bowel, this means that there is nothing pathological that medical science can find in the structure of your bowel. Despite the absence of structural problems, the functioning of your bowel is disturbed and you may have, among other symptoms, spasm, pain, bloating, constipation, diarrhea, and the increased anxiety connected with these symptoms.

There are many books on each of the disorders discussed below, including discussions of their anatomy, physiology, psychology, causes, as well as various treatment options. My purpose here is to identify conditions that may be helped using *Paradoxical Relaxation* as well as discuss some special requirements in the treatment of specific disorders. I briefly discuss each of these disorders and how *Paradoxical Relaxation* might be particularly useful for them, as well as briefly discussing other complementary interventions that I have seen to be helpful. My disclaimer here is that the information here is not meant to substitute for medical or psychiatric evaluation and treatment. Learning *Paradoxical Relaxation* should be done with a health care provider competent in *Paradoxical Relaxation.*

> Somatization is a name given to the psychophysical process in which physical symptoms are triggered by emotional or mental factors like anxiety

I use the term somatization to refer to the phenomenon of emotional disturbance causing physical symptoms. The idea behind the word is that what is emotional or mental is somehow transformed into something somatic or physical. Examples of somatization include muscle related pelvic pain, anxiety triggered heartburn, non-cardiac chest pain, gastrointestinal spasm and pain usually called irritable bowel syndrome or idiopathic dyspepsia, headache, low back pain, constipation, insomnia, heart palpitations and arrhythmia, and jaw pain from teeth grinding among other kinds of symptoms. Somatization, which produces physical symptoms, is sometimes understood to *bind* anxiety—that is to say, it gives a person a place to tie up or bind what is otherwise free-floating anxiety. In an unexpected way, turning anxiety into physical symptoms can stabilize and lower anxiety by turning it into a physical condition. It has been my observation that the level of anxiety often reduces, though certainly does not go away, as the person's focus of anxiety shifts to the physical condition.

John Sarno, through his work with back pain, is a compelling advocate of the connection between emotional disturbance translating into physical symptoms. In his best-selling books *Mind Over Back Pain, The Mind-Body Prescription,* and *Healing Back Pain: The Mind-Body Connection,* he proposes that most back pain exists as the way people distract themselves from their emotional and interpersonal problems. He treats patients with what he calls "tension myositis syndrome" by having them focus on the emotional and interpersonal parts of their lives, instead of focusing on their physical symptoms.

## Symptoms substitution: when one physical symptom gets better and is substituted by another

There are times when physical symptoms triggered by anxiety migrate from one part of the body to another. At other times, when the person is no longer troubled by the physical symptoms, anxiety that has been free-floating comes back. *Paradoxical Relaxation* is an important practice because it can lower the arousal of the nervous system whether the nervous system arousal is triggering physical symptoms or simply producing the experience of free-floating anxiety. The skill of being able to calm down a nervous system that is aroused and upset is the key issue here, more significant and therapeutic than simply resolving physical symptoms which can migrate from one part of the body to another.

## Example of the mechanism of somatization: a *tail-pulled-between-the-legs*, anxiety, and pelvic pain

How does anxiety turn into physical symptoms? In the following discussion of the *tail-pulled-between-the-legs*, I want to describe one pathway in which I understand how fear is translated into physical symptoms.

Looking at the functional disorder of pelvic pain is instructive in beginning to see one mechanism of muscle tightening and the production of somatic symptoms in response to anxiety. Here is a compelling view of the relationship of chronic anxiety, pelvic pain, and the biological reaction of mammals to pull their tail between their legs when threatened.

## Pulling the tail between the legs in mammals as a response of fear

It is common knowledge that a dog will pull his tail between his legs when he is fearful. Other emotions have been attributed to this *tail-pulled-between-the-legs* behavior including shame, dread, defeat or shyness. For the present discussion, I submit here that the root emotion for this *tail-pulled-between-the-legs* behavior is fear.

In the typology of Walter Cannon, the great Harvard physiologist of the early 20$^{th}$ century who introduced the phrase *fight, flight, freeze* to describe the varieties of survival behavior in mammals, a *tail-pulled-between-the-legs* is an expression of the survival behavior *freeze*. This *freeze* behavior expresses the organism's attempt to self-protectively hold fast waiting for danger to pass. The behavior of a waving tail, on the other hand, has been associated among animal watchers with the emotions of excitement, happiness, or aggression, contrasting sharply to the *tail-pulled-between-the-legs*-behavior. Most cat and dog owners intuitively read their animals' behavior, in large part, by what the tail is doing.

In humans, the tailbone is commonly understood to be what remains of the tail in our humanoid ancestors. This tailbone (coccyx) is sometimes called the vestigial tail. In humans, the *coccygeal, iliococcygeal and pubococcygeal* muscles of the pelvic basin are attached to the coccyx or tailbone and are responsible for its movement. The phenomenon of pulling the tail between the legs uses the *coccygeal, iliococcygeal and pubococcygeal muscles (and other muscles attached and connected to the tailbone*) to protect the body from a perceived threat. In this act of muscle activity, the *coccygeal, iliococcygeal, pubococcygeal* muscles contract, causing the tail to pull in.

## Anxiety is intimately related to the biological reflex of pulling the tail between the legs

To my knowledge, in the scientific discussion of pelvic pain in general, or somatization in particular, there has not been a discussion of what I believe to be the intimate relationship between *tail-pulled-between-the-legs* behavior and pelvic pain. Here I introduce this idea and the therapeutic implications of this unlikely and yet clinically important relationship.

From the beginning of our research at Stanford with pelvic pain, our premise has been that the functional disorder of pelvic pain, pelvic pain in which no physical pathology could be found, was related to chronic self-protective muscle contraction that triggered a self-feeding cycle of tension, anxiety, pain, and protective guarding. In the original publication of our book, *A Headache in the Pelvis,* we summarized our understanding as follows:

> *We have identified a group of chronic pelvic pain syndromes that we believe is caused by the overuse of the human instinct to protect the genitals, rectum, and contents of the pelvis from injury or pain by contracting the pelvic muscles. This tendency becomes exaggerated in predisposed individuals and over time results in chronic pelvic pain and dysfunction. The state of chronic constriction creates pain-referring trigger points, reduced blood flow, and an inhospitable environment for the nerves, blood vessels, and structures*

> *throughout the pelvic basin. This results in a cycle of tension, anxiety, and pain, which has previously been unrecognized and untreated.*
>
> *Understanding this tension, anxiety, and pain cycle has allowed us to create an effective treatment. Our program breaks the cycle by rehabilitating the shortened pelvic muscles and connective tissue supporting the pelvic organs while simultaneously using a specific methodology to modify the tendency to tighten the muscles of the pelvic floor under stress.*

Pulling the tail between the legs is a mammalian self-protective reflex occurring both in mammals with tails, and mammals, like humans, with vestigial tails, otherwise known as tailbones. I am proposing that much pelvic pain in humans occurs when, in states of intense or ongoing anxiety, individuals chronically pull their 'tail' between their legs. In fact, the muscular activity of pulling the 'tail' between the legs contracts the pelvic floor muscles, and if done chronically, causes a painful shortening and contraction of the coccygeal muscles as they pull the tailbone (tail) in. Upon examination, these muscles are among the most commonly trigger-pointed muscles in patients with pelvic pain. In our recently published study mapping trigger points in patients with pelvic pain, the coccygeus muscles were among the most common muscles to be symptomatic and painful.

## The somatization of anxiety into muscle-related pelvic pain can come from a universal, biologically-based event

In this example I am offering a description of somatization, focusing on the link between anxiety and the physical expression of anxiety in a functional disorder. I am suggesting here that certain kinds of pelvic pain come from a universal, biologically- based event that appears hardwired in mammals. This event is essentially invisible to us in our fellow humans because we humans do not have a tail to inform others of our states of fear and anxiety. In other words, I am suggesting that muscle-related pelvic pain is a chronic *tail-pulled-between-the legs* syndrome. It involves various chronically contracted muscles that tighten the *entire* pelvic floor, and the ongoing symptoms of this condition are fed by tension, anxiety, pain and protective guarding.

## The problem in the effective and coordinated treatment of functional disorders when they cross traditional lines of medical sub-specialization

When someone has an anxiety-related disorder, most people don't have a doctor who understands and coordinates all medical and non-medical aspects of the treatment. At this time in health care specialization, most health care practitioners stay within the traditional bounds of their sub-specialization and it is unusual that they coordinate their patients' treatments with those of practitioners in other sub-specialties who are essential for effective treatment. The treatment of anxiety-related disorders is cross-disciplinary. At this time in the history of medicine, few sub-specialties treats functional disorders with the the kinds of interventions required.

For instance, if you have irritable bowel syndrome, the gastroenterologist will likely perform tests to make the diagnosis and suggest diet modifications, the addition of fiber, stool softeners or laxatives, and perhaps some medication to quiet down an irritated bowel. A good gastroenterologist will probably suggest stress reduction and refer you to someone who offers that service. He might recommend a dietician for nutritional counseling.

Typically, the person who teaches stress reduction or nutritional counseling pays little attention to the issues addressed by the gastroenterologist. Often patients are then left to fend for themselves, trying to coordinate all of the components together coherently. I want to offer this section from the perspective of a coordinator of treatment who has a wide view of the treatment that includes both relaxation and non-relaxation components and the coordination of these components.

## Functional Disorders that may be helped by *Paradoxical Relaxation*

Here are a list of functional disorders that may be helped by *Paradoxical Relaxation*:

- Constipation, anal fissures and hemorrhoids
- Irritable bowel syndrome (IBS)
- Hypertension (high blood pressure)
- Insomnia
- Headaches
- Temporomandibular Disorders (TMD/TMJ)
- Jaw-tension related tinnitus (ringing in the ears)
- Cardiac Arryhthmia

*Paradoxical Relaxation* was originally developed as part of the *Wise-Anderson Protocol* designed to help patients calm down or resolve their chronic pelvic pain related to chronically tightened muscles in the pelvis. Using *Paradoxical Relaxation* in a modified *Wise-Anderson Protocol* may be helpful in treating these other functional somatic disorders.

## Using Trigger Point Release, stretching, and hot baths in conjunction with *Paradoxical Relaxation* for functional disorders

In our work with pelvic pain we have found it helpful that before engaging in the practice of calming down the body and mind using *Paradoxical Relaxation*, the patient stretch the specific muscles. While yoga postures are an excellent form of stretching, I believe that the self-treatment physical therapy of *Trigger Point Release* is more specific and can be more effective.

## The best order: physical exercise, hot bath, *Trigger Point Release,* stretching, and lastly *Paradoxical Relaxation*

In our work with pelvic pain we have found that physical self-treatment including trigger point release developed by Travell and Simons, skin rolling and certain kinds of stretching before relaxation tends to make the relaxation session easier and more effective. In the *Wise-Anderson Protocol* for pelvic pain, we recommend that when possible, the patient do some form of aerobic exercise for a period of 20-45 minutes, followed by a 5-15 minute hot bath, followed by *Trigger Point Release* and stretching, followed by 25-45 minutes of *Paradoxical Relaxation.*

The time commitment it takes to do all of this is obviously not trivial and it is not always possible to devote this kind of time to treating a functional disorder. Nevertheless, unless setting aside this kind of time is the rule rather than the exception, any real results are unlikely to occur.

It is advisable to have at least one session of *Trigger Point Release* done by a competent physical therapist or expert in *Trigger Point Release. The Trigger Point Therapy Workbook* by Clair Davies, in my opinion, is the best self-help book for external *Trigger Point Release.*

## Constipation, anal fissures, and hemorrhoids

Strictly speaking, anal fissures and hemorrhoids are not functional disorders because they are observable disturbances in the physical structure of the body. The anal fissure manifests as a tear in the anus and hemorrhoids manifest as a kind of varicose vein, which tends to balloon out when straining on the toilet. I include them here because they are psychosomatic conditions often triggered by anxiety and can be helped with the reduction of anxiety.

The colon and rectum operate together in the activity of the evacuation of stool. Normal bowel elimination involves a complex mechanism which includes the reflex relaxation of the internal anal sphincter when the rectum is full. This sensory muscle, which is autonomically controlled, can differentiate between gas or stool and signal the pelvic floor muscles to relax if it is appropriate to eliminate (along with appropriate peristalsis in the colon). However, if it is not socially appropriate or convenient, an individual can voluntarily tighten up the pelvic floor and help quiet down the sense of urgency that is felt.

Heightened anxiety can lead to increased tension in the pelvic floor. This can interfere with the ability of the muscles to release at the appropriate time, at the same time can disturb normal peristalsis in the bowel. There are also individuals who have learned to do the opposite of what needs to be done in order to eliminate. Instead of relaxing their pelvic floor muscles, especially the pubo-rectalis muscle, they contract their muscles while attempting to eliminate, causing a frustrating condition called paradoxical puborectalis contraction. Fortunately, this condition is relatively easily diagnosed, and reversible with neuro-muscular re-education. It is important to stop the habit of this paradoxical contraction, as prolonged bearing down can result in prolapsing pelvic or abdominal organs.

The anal fissure is like a paper cut in the mucosal lining of the anal sphincter. It is understood by many researchers that the anal fissure is called an *ischemic ulcer*. Ischemia is a condition in which there is a significant reduction in blood flow to an area. The current understanding about anal fissures is that because there is elevated tension, the blood flow in the anal sphincter is reduced, making the tissue fragile and reducing the opening of the sphincter which then becomes vulnerable to injury from a hard bowel movement and from the pressure of bearing down during defecation.

It is generally agreed that the source of the anal fissure in large part involves a chronically tightened internal anal sphincter. Both surgery, the procedure of stretching or dilating the anal sphincter under anesthesia, and the application of topical agents to the internal anal sphincter are aimed at relaxing the anal sphincter. The surgical concept for anal fissures is based on the peculiar idea that cutting the sphincter is the best way to reduce the tone, tension, and spasm in the anal sphincter. While surgery is often successful, there is risk of short-term and sometimes long-term fecal incontinence.

At some time or another, many people find a little blood in their stool, usually after a particularly hard bowel movement. One can become confused and upset at such an event. At other times, alarmed individuals go to the doctor complaining of rectal pain after a bowel movement with no apparent blood in the stool. Often the doctor gives the diagnosis of anal fissure or hemorrhoids to these complaints. Hemorrhoids constitute another condition that is painful and sometimes the source of blood in the stool.

## Conventional treatment of constipation, anal fissures, and hemorrhoids tends to ignore the relationship between body and mind

The conventional medical treatment of constipation, anal fissures, and hemorrhoids tends to ignore the relationship between mind and body. Like the conventional treatment of pelvic pain, the relationship of a person's mindset, level of relaxation during bowel movements, and management of stress is almost entirely ignored in the literature on the treatment of constipation, anal fissures, and hemorrhoids. Instead, there is a narrow focus on immediately reducing symptoms of these conditions. Medications and sometimes surgery are the usual options.

In the case of anal fissures and hemorrhoids, most of the patients we have seen who have had surgery reported that the physicians they saw offered few options related to quieting down the anxiety and habitual straining and tightening related to these conditions. Instead of seeing an anal fissure as an expression of anxiety and chronic pelvic tension, conventional treatment sees its symptoms, including chronic anal tension, as something that needs to be mechanically or pharmaceutically stopped. Little regard is shown for the big picture of a person's life and how one's symptoms are a response to this big picture. It is my view that the symptom is the way our bodies are trying to communicate. If we refuse to understand the message because we don't understand the body's language, we needlessly suffer and don't deal with the root problem prompting the symptom.

In the large majority of cases, it is the chronic tension in the pelvic floor, including the anal sphincter, usually combined with diet, anxiety and time urgency around bowel habits that strongly contributes to constipation, anal fissures, and hemorrhoids. The chronic pelvic tension, diet, and bowel habits associated with most constipation, anal fissures and hemorrhoids do not come out of the blue. In a word, a person's mind, body, and lifestyle are involved in the creation and perpetuation of these conditions.

In our book *A Headache in the Pelvis,* we proposed that a modified *Wise-Anderson Protocol* might be of significant benefit for the treatment of constipation, anal fissures, and hemorrhoids. The overriding principle is that these conditions tend to occur as the result of anxiety and someone expressing this anxiety by tightening in the pelvic floor and in the case of constipation, inhibiting normal peristaltic movement in the colon. Where sphincterotomy, or the partial cutting of the internal anal sphincter, to reduce anal sphincter tension is often used for anal fissures, I believe that it is often possible to learn to relax the anal sphincter with no surgery. This may be accomplished by teaching patients the *Trigger Point Release* and *Paradoxical Relaxation* protocols we use for pelvic pain syndromes. A devoted effort of self-treatment in the *Wise-Anderson Protocol* that we teach in our 6-day clinics for pelvic pain would be more than sufficient training for someone suffering from constipation, anal fissures, and hemorrhoids. Of course, the modification of the protocol would have to include diet and bathroom habit re-education, such as teaching the patient not to strain unduly, and not to resist the feeling of urgency to go to the bathroom.

## Irritable bowel syndrome (IBS)

IBS is common in the general population and is reputed to account for up to 50% of visits to gastroenterologists. The symptoms of IBS typically include, among other symptoms: abdominal pain, abdominal bloating or fullness, diarrhea or constipation, sometimes heartburn, early feelings of fullness and incomplete bowel emptying. Typically it is treated with certain medications, avoiding colon irritating food and drink, increasing intake of water and fiber and exercise. It is a distressing but not malignant disorder, and it often comes and goes with periods of stress.

## Spastic esophagus and globus hystericus

The esophagus is a muscular structure that transports food from the mouth to the stomach through the rhythmic peristaltic movement of the esophageal muscles. In certain individuals, the esophagus can go into spasm. This spasm can delay the transport of food and cause chest pain that is often misdiagnosed as angina. When not confused with heart related chest pain, it is sometimes called non-cardiac chest pain. There is a form of esophageal spasm called *globus hystericus* or more recently called *globus pharyngis* which is commonly felt as a 'lump in the throat'. People with globus hystericus often try to persistently clear their throat and rid themselves of the sensation that something is caught in the throat. The 'lump in the throat' can be caused by inflammation but is often caused by anxiety. The people I have treated with globus hystericus have often had a sense of wanting to cry but not being able to. The psychology of globus hystericus, in my experience, often involves the suppression of emotion.

My teacher Edmund Jacobson was often successful in patients with esophageal spasm and globus hystericus. He did x-ray evaluations of the spastic esophagus before and after relaxation treatment and the x-ray showed a dramatic relaxation of the esophagus. Many cases of esophageal spasm, I believe can be helped by lowering nervous system arousal.

## Using *Paradoxical Relaxation* and a modified *Wise-Anderson Protocol* for the treatment of irritable bowel syndrome, esophageal spasm, and globus hystericus.

In our 6-day pelvic pain clinics, some patients who also suffer from irritable bowel syndrome and/or have reported improvement in their IBS and ER symptoms. These patients have reported that this improvement occurred after doing abdominal *Trigger Point Release* followed by *Paradoxical Relaxation.*

IBS is common with both male and female patients whom we have treated for pelvic pain. Because the purpose of the *Wise-Anderson Protocol* is to teach patients targeted self-treatment methods, one of the methods we show patients is abdominal *Trigger Point Release.* In some pelvic pain patients with IBS, their symptoms of abdominal discomfort sometimes improved when they exerted *Trigger Point Release*-type pressure to most areas of tenderness or pain throughout their abdomen. When this intervention was effective, they found that the discomfort sometimes dissipated. This was done in conjunction with the regular practice of *Paradoxical Relaxation.*

The areas palpated tended to center around the ascending, transverse, and descending colon and the area around the lower esophageal sphincter. Patients practiced relaxation simultaneously while doing pressure release in these areas. In other words, while they were pressing on uncomfortable abdominal areas, they consciously relaxed. Anyone who wishes to do this should only only attempt this under the guidance of a physician.

In their classic book *The Colon*, Stewart Wolf and Harold G. Wolff observed that in patients with abdominal fistulas (open holes in the abdomen) that permitted direct visual examination of the colon in different emotional states, the colons of subjects studied tended to become slowed down and contracted (hypodynamic)—- stopping their rhythmic movement—during periods of fear, dejection, futility or defeat, dissatisfaction, boredom, tension and mild depression. The subjects' colons became hyperactive (hyperdynamic) in moments of anger, resentment, guilt, humiliation, anxiety and conflict. When the emotional states of these individuals became quiet and undistressed, the colonic behavior normalized and the rhythmic peristaltic movement resumed. The visual examination of the colon is rare and the observations of Wolf and Wolff are precious and offer insight into what goes on in the colon in relationship to emotions.

> *"In the patients described it was common to find a disturbance of colonic function characterized either by a hyperdynamic response with diarrhea, or a hypodynamic response with constipation. Hyper-function was characterized by hyperemia, a contraction of longitudinal muscles together*

> *with shortening of the colon and increase in rhythmic contractile activity of circular muscles in the caecum, ascending, and transverse loops while the descending and sigmoid colon showed no rhythmic circular contractions but assumed a rigid tubular shape due to longitudinal muscle activity, with pallor of the mucosa. In colonic hypofunction with constipation, rectal, anal and perianal muscles were usually contracted so as to further impede emptying....The hypodynamic reaction was encountered when individuals reacted...with feelings of fear, dejection, futility, or defeat, dissatisfaction, boredom, tension and mild depression... sustained or recurrent colonic hypofunction in patients was found to be associated with constipation... may be looked upon as a part of a general reaction of 'grimly holding fast' under circumstances that threatened the individual. The hyperdynamic reaction of the colon, on the other hand... (was related to) symbolic assaults which included anger, resentment, guilt, humiliation, anxiety and conflict. Catastrophic or shocking situations or those arousing feelings of being overwhelmed also evoked hyperfunction of the large bowel... (this can be called) the ejection-riddance pattern of colonic hyperfunction."*

## Hypertension (high blood pressure)

Hypertension refers to excessive pressure on the walls of the blood vessels in the body. Hypertension is a big subject and has a number of different causes. Some forms of hypertension, however, can be exacerbated by stress. There has been considerable research published on the efficacy of using biofeedback in reducing blood pressure. Lowering autonomic arousal and calming down anxiety using relaxation may help a certain group of people with hypertension.

## Insomnia

People who suffer from chronic anxiety symptoms commonly struggle with insomnia. Whether it is anxiety, continual pain, or nocturnal urinary frequency and urgency, many of our patients describe the havoc of being awakened several times during the night, not being able to fall back to sleep, and not getting a good night's rest.

Edmund Jacobson remarked that the quality of relaxation during the day tends to determine the quality of sleep at night. *Paradoxical Relaxation* can help with both the difficulty of falling asleep as well as with the difficulty of going back to sleep after one has awakened. Until all symptoms are *substantially* reduced, however, a good night's sleep can remain problematic.

Falling asleep tends to be easier to solve than going back to sleep, but we can help our patients with both difficulties. The help that *Paradoxical Relaxation* can offer in falling asleep is simple. If you have any facility in *Paradoxical Relaxation*, there is usually a high likelihood that doing this relaxation will enable you to fall asleep more easily.

## The difficulty of falling asleep

What typically keeps you from falling asleep at night, barring a nervous system jolted by coffee or other stimulants, is your mind flitting from one thought to another. Training your attention to rest in sensation can essentially stop this mind flitting and help reduce the arousal of your nervous system. It is much easier to fall asleep when you are able to stop your mind from darting here and there. Using *Paradoxical Relaxation* to fall asleep by focusing attention on sensation and returning attention remorselessly when it wanders can help the problem of going to sleep. It is often possible to be able to fall asleep in a relatively short amount of time after practicing in *Paradoxical Relaxation* for a few months.

## Sleep can be more anxiety-producing than being awake

Some chronically anxious people find themselves more anxious at night and when they are dreaming. They feel no control over the images in their dreams that are often distressing and around which they feel helpless.

The sense of helplessness is perhaps what is most difficult to deal with when one has distressing dreams. Many anxious people have made a point of creating a life in which they are productive and feel in charge. When they are productive and feel in charge, their anxiety reduces. At a certain level, being competent, successful and in control is an anti-anxiety strategy for someone who is chronically anxious. It is a way of reassuring the frightened child inside that everything is okay. In sleep, these anxious people become subject to their dream images and don't have the experience of being in charge and in control and this is why they often are more anxious sleeping than being awake.

## Going back to sleep

When we awake in the middle of the night, it tends to be more difficult to go back to sleep. For this reason, we suggest that when you cannot go back to sleep, you get up and wake yourself. Sometimes splashing water on your face or walking briefly around the house can help.

Upon awakening, some patients have found it useful to do the yoga-like stretches and other methods they have learned in the *Trigger Point Release* sessions. In addition to these exercises, specific yoga stretches sometimes can help relax the body. These stretches can take between five minutes to half an hour. Some patients go back to sleep using the current relaxation lesson they are doing. This relaxation can be done in bed.

## Not making insomnia an enemy

From time to time when I have had sleep disturbance, I have remembered the words of one of my gestalt therapy teachers, Jim Simkin, who used to say: "Insomnia is nothing to lose sleep over." I took what he said to mean that it was easier to go back to sleep if you didn't make insomnia, into something about which to be anxious.

This insight has served me. I usually have no trouble falling asleep. At times I wake up in the middle of the night and I have come to regard this waking up with equanimity. In knowing that I can fall back to sleep using *Paradoxical Relaxation*, I have used this middle-of-the-night-time to write, read, do work, or take a hot bath for an hour or so. I have come to appreciate that this is a time that is always quiet and undisturbed, when I have nothing else pulling me. If I find myself waking up in the middle of the night, any writing or work I do tends to be productive and going back to sleep after being up for a little while tends to be easy using the relaxation method in this book.

*The key to falling asleep is to completely accept the feeling of being awake while practicing Paradoxical Relaxation to go back to sleep.* When I first attempted to use relaxation to go back to sleep, I subtly inwardly resisted the feeling of being awake which was the result of my nervous system being aroused. I resisted my arousal, in a sense tried to deny it and subtly forced down my inward feeling of being amped up. Again, this resistance was subtle.

Now I don't resist being aroused. I do my best to completely accept my feeling of being amped up. So when I find myself not sleepy at all, I lie there completely accepting my feeling of being awake as I rest my attention in the sensation of some tension I feel. And lo and behold, I usually conk out in a few minutes.

## Transforming early morning anxiety into your muse

How do you transform your early morning anxiety into your muse? The word 'muse' was originally used in 1374 to mean protector of the arts, from the Greek *mousa* meaning muse, music, song. A muse is generally thought of as that which inspires creativity.

You can use your early morning anxious awakening as your muse, as your inspiration for getting things done, especially things involving creativity. Transforming early morning anxiety into a muse is counter-intuitive when you are under the sheets of a warm bed and are tired and wanting simply to be asleep.

It is common for anxious people in general and our pelvic pain patients in particular to wake up anxious. Often this waking up with anxiety occurs quite early in the morning. Rodney Anderson's Stanford study of male pelvic pain patients showed a precipitous rise in cortisol in the morning in men suffering with chronic pelvic pain syndrome. Cortisol rise in the morning is a common phenomenon of anxious people in general and I believe that this steep rise in cortisol in our pelvic pain patients is intimately associated with their tendency toward anxiety.

It is not uncommon for anxious people who wake up with anxiety to remain in bed in a groggy and half-awake state during these periods of early morning anxiety. Few like to get out of a warm bed when they are sleepy early in the morning, even if they do experience anxiety.

*Generally, staying in bed in the half-awake state during early morning bouts of anxiety is not productive for a number of reasons.* Staying in a half awake state of anxiety usually results in neither being able to have the benefit of falling back to sleep, nor the productiveness of waking up. While *Paradoxical Relaxation* is often able to help calm down this kind of anxiety, it is more difficult to use *Paradoxical Relaxation* to do this when you are half awake and anxious during the early-morning cortisol storm that tends to plague anxious people.

You can get the most benefit from *Paradoxical Relaxation* when you are awake, have presence of mind and the energy to focus your attention. Doing *Paradoxical Relaxation* at a time when your nervous system has calmed down is far better than doing it in the midst of cortisol-related anxiety.

During the anxious period that typically occurs upon awakening, you can spend the cortisol-driven energy working on a report, cleaning the house, painting a picture, writing a story, or involving yourself in some other project or creative enterprise. The morning *anxiety state* enables sustained and energetic focus and some people do the best work of the day off of the energy of cortisol that is secreted in the early morning when the whole world is still asleep and you are undisturbed.

After an hour or so of this kind of activity, the disturbance of the early morning *anxiety state* tends to abate. Doing *Paradoxical Relaxation* becomes much easier and more effective. Once the cortisol is 'spent' in the completion of creative projects or work projects, *Paradoxical Relaxation* is much easier and you can often use it to get the most delicious and relaxed sleep after 'spending' the cortisol boost on something productive rather than simply suffering from it.

An important aspect of making anxiety your muse in early morning awakening is to abandon any thoughts of guilt, shame, sense of I-shouldn't-be up-now, or feeling badly in any way about being up at such a time. The attitude instead should be along the lines of: "I am doing my very best with my anxiety now and this will make it much more likely that when I get back to sleep, I will be able to sleep much more deeply. In the meantime, it isn't bad that I am getting something done."

## Headache

Headaches can be a symptom for a number of problems and the headaches helped by relaxation are headaches where there is no pathological disorder nor structural problem (where the headache is not indicative of some other condition).

Relaxation of the muscle tension associated with headaches as well as reducing nervous system arousal can be helpful in reducing the frequency, intensity, and incidence of certain kinds of headaches.

## Temporomandibular Disorders (TMD/TMJ)

Temporomandibular disorder is the name given to jaw pain or pain in the temporomandibular joint which connects the lower jaw to the temporal bone of the skull. This is a joint that allows the jaw to move smoothly up and down and side to side. This is the muscle that is tightened when you clench your jaw. When we were writing the book *A Headache in the Pelvis,* one of the titles we considered was *TMJ of the Pelvis* because the jaw (along with the abdomen and pelvis) is one of the places that people commonly tighten up or clench when they are anxious. When we did an informal study of jaw tension and pelvic floor tension at Stanford, we found that when the jaw relaxed (as measured by electromyography) the pelvic floor simultaneously relaxed.

While the literature about TMD tends not to focus on the primary stress relationship between anxiety and stress and the occurrence of TMD, I am clear that most of TMD has to do with anxiety and the body protectively guarding in the way that I have described in this book. The jaw happens to be one of the very clear places that you can clench when you are anxious. Teeth grinding at night does not happen to someone who, in my opinion, is relaxed and happy. Teeth grinding happens when you are aroused and guarding yourself.

The typical treatment for TMD by dentists involves having the patient wear some kind of mouth guard during sleep so that the teeth are protected and not worn down or injured. While that is very important in terms of dental health, it doesn't address the real problem. It doesn't address the problem at all of the stress and anxiety that is promoting the chronic tightening of the jaw.

A small, unpublished study done in the 1980's had the remarkable result of reducing nighttime teeth grinding by simply reminding people to relax their jaw with a device called a Motiv-Aider (a device mentioned previously in this book, which can be useful in doing *Moment-to-Moment Relaxation*). The Motiv-Aider vibrated at frequent intervals throughout the day to remind the teeth-grinding patient to relax their jaw at the moment the Motiv-Aider was vibrating. When they relaxed their jaw every time the Motiv-Aider went off, and stopped tightening the jaw for two weeks during the study, there was an astonishing drop in nighttime teeth grinding.

This was a kind of behavior modification method to help relax the tendency to grind teeth. When someone has tightened their jaw repetitively, the muscles shorten and trigger points form. As a way of restoring the pain-free state of the jaw, trigger point therapy can be very helpful. The trigger points that are involved in TMD are relatively straight-forward and an explanation for their proper deactivation can be found in the Clair Davies book mentioned previously (*The Trigger Point Therapy Workbook*).

This form of relaxation is related to what we discussed in *A Headache in the Pelvis* (and previously in this book) as *Moment-to-Moment Relaxation. Moment-to-Moment Relaxation* can be used to help calm down the tendency to tighten up in all of the areas of the body, not just the jaw. Doing *Paradoxical Relaxation* for TMD should begin with the relaxation of the forehead, neck, or shoulders for a number of weeks before attempting relaxation of the jaw itself. Relaxation of the jaw can be a challenge because the jaw can remain very tight for an extended period of time and having patience in allowing it to be tight requires some practice in *Paradoxical Relaxation*. Furthermore, the jaw will tend to relax more when the forehead, which typically is an easier place to relax, is quiet.

## Tinnitus (ringing in the ears)

Tinnitus can involve a chronic high-pitched whistling, ringing, buzzing sound in the ears and can have a number of causes. If you have this symptom, it is obviously something that would be appropriate to see an ear-nose-throat doctor about. *Paradoxical Relaxation* has been able to reduce or resolve a very specific kind of tinnitus having to do with jaw tension. When there is no structural abnormality and no physical reason can be found for it, *Paradoxical Relaxation* is a benign treatment for this certain kind of tinnitus. The relaxation of the jaw and *Trigger Point Release* in and around the jaw may be helpful for this kind of tinnitus.

## Cardiac Arrhythmia

By lowering the baseline level of anxiety and autonomic arousal, *Paradoxical Relaxation* may be able to reduce certain kinds of anxiety-related cardiac arrhythmias, particularly arrhythmias related to palpitations, ectopic beats, preventricular contractions (PVC's), or atrial ventricular contractions (AVC's). Anxiety can exacerbate or set off these disturbances in the rhythm of the heart.

Normally the heart beats regularly with a regular change in intervals between beats and inhalation and exhalation occur. When adrenaline is pumped into the system, the heart rate can increase. When someone is in an *anxiety state* or in panic, disturbing palpitations can occur. Palpitations can feel like something has dropped inside your chest, or that your heart has skipped a beat. This often happens in normal people, when they have a skipped heartbeat now and again. When these skipped heartbeats occur regularly they can be disturbing.

For individuals who have what is called lone paroxysmal atrial fibrillation, their heart beats normally but some kind of stress can trigger their heart to beat irregularly. These individuals are often advised to avoid what agitates their nervous system including the avoidance of caffeine, alcohol, and certain kinds of drugs.

Keeping the nervous system quiet can help reduce the triggering of atrial fibrillation. Regular *Paradoxical Relaxation* along with other lifestyle changes that calm down nervous system arousal may help someone who has a tendency toward atrial fibrillation under stress to reduce the frequency of such episodes.

# Chapter 16

## *Conclusion*

This book represents my attempt to express what I have learned over the years in regularly practicing *Paradoxical Relaxation* as well as in teaching *Paradoxical Relaxation* to others. Maintaining any equanimity in my own life is not a simple matter. Like most of us, I have many stresses with which I deal. Yet I can say that I am able, using this method, to come back into peace much of the time I choose to.

What I write in this book may not mean very much to someone who has never brought their attention inside and worked with themselves to calm down their agitation and anxiety. I think this book will mean more to someone who has been doing *Paradoxical Relaxation* or some related method because what I say here comes from what I believe to be universal principles from which all relaxation and meditation methods borrow. This universal principle is that only through ending all resistance to what is happening that cannot be changed in the moment can we enter the gateway of inner peace.

As I look at this book, I see very clearly that the heart of what I want to present in the method of *Paradoxical Relaxation* is the *how to* of *giving it up to get it (*as much as it is possible to ever teach that). I do this as a student myself of this method. Specifically, I discuss the acceptance of anxiety and tension in order to relax them. Beyond that, I am sharing my own experience that the fastest way to resolve all the things that feels adverse, uncomfortable, and unpleasant inside, after I have actively done everything I can to deal with them, is to *have a practice* of accepting them.

There is very little bang for the buck in simply knowing the concept of accepting what you want to let go of. My major point in this book is that getting good at such acceptance is not inborn, but instead requires repeated, disciplined practice. This is the same kind of practice required to get good at playing the violin or playing tennis. Accepting everything inside means saying *yes* to the subtlest and what have often been the most unconscious of feelings, sensations, and inner activities. It is perhaps the most profound existential skill anyone can develop.

David Wise
Sebastopol, California

# Chapter 17

*Contact*

## Training in *Paradoxical Relaxation*

I am primarily involved in the treatment of pelvic pain using the *Wise-Anderson Protocol.* From time to time, I offer trainings in *Paradoxical Relaxation.*


### Contact information

**Telephone**: 707 874 2225

**Fax** 707 874 2335

**Email**: ahip@sonic.net

**Mailing address**: PO Box 54
Occidental, California 95465

**Website**: www.pelvicpainhelp.com

## About the Author

David Wise, Ph.D. worked at Stanford University as a Research Scholar in the department of Urology for 8 years where he co-developed with Dr. Rodney Anderson, the *Wise-Anderson Protocol* (popularly called the *Stanford Protocol*), a new treatment for pelvic pain syndromes in men and women. He is the coauthor of the book *A Headache in the Pelvis: A New Understanding and Treatment for Chronic Pelvic Pain Syndromes*. He has been a plenary speaker at the National Institutes of Health, and published and presented research on the *Wise-Anderson Protocol*. His major professional interests have been in autonomic self-regulation, functional somatic disorders, transpersonal psychotherapy, and the psychology of the creative process.

He is a painter and sculptor and enjoys drawing in cafes. He has done carpentry and woodworking for many years. He plays the piano, guitar, and mandolin and has written several musical plays. He played in a klezmer band and for many years played popular Italian music and opera at Caffe Trieste in San Francisco. He has made a number of musical albums including *The Music of Segal and Wise, Life in the Slow Lane, The Yiddish Favorites of Sam Wise, Songs From a Course in Miracles,* and *San Francisco, San Francisco.* He lives in northern California.

## Disclaimer

The information contained in this book is not meant to substitute for competent medical or psychological evaluation or treatment. With any physical condition or psychological condition, one should consult with a physician or psychologist before initiating any strategy of treatment including the use of *Paradoxical Relaxation.*